# Parent Medication Checklist

BEFORE GIVING your child ANY medication make sure that the following questions are answered and understood.

- ☐ What is the medicine's name?
- ☐ What does it do?
- ☐ How much do I give?
- ☐ How often must I give it?
- ☐ How long do I need to continue giving the medicine?
- ☐ Are there special preparation instructions; do I need to shake it vigorously?
- ☐ Are there special times to take the medicine?
- ☐ Must I refrigerate the medicine?
- ☐ Are there common side effects I can expect?
- ☐ Are there rare adverse risks that I should be aware of?
- ☐ If my child has a known allergy, might he/she also be allergic to this drug?
- ☐ How much does this medicine cost?
- ☐ Is a generic form of comparable quality available?

**FINALLY**

- ☐ Is this medicine really needed? Do the benefits outweigh the risks and costs?

# The Parent's Pharmacy

*Preventing and Treating Childhood Illnesses*

Robert H. Pantell, M.D., and David A. Bergman, M.D.

**ADDISON-WESLEY PUBLISHING COMPANY**
*Reading, Massachusetts • Menlo Park, California • London
Amsterdam • Don Mills, Ontario • Sydney*

**Library of Congress Cataloging in Publication Data**

Pantell, Robert H., 1945–
   The parent's pharmacy.


   Includes index.
      1. Drugs—Popular works. 2. Therapeutics—Popular works. 3. Pediatric
pharmacology. I. Bergman, David, 1946–     . II. Title.
RJ560.P36   1982                615.5'8'0240431                82-13837
ISBN 0-201-08153-9
ISBN 0-201-08154-7 (pbk.)

*To Parents*
**Who keep their children healthy**
*by caring for them*
*by showing them how to care for themselves &*
*by teaching us.*

# Acknowledgments

THIS WORK was helped enormously by the support of our families. Thanks, Aaron, Annie, Gretchen, Maureen, Peter, Phred, and Sophie.

Numerous colleagues provided feedback. Wayne Weart, Pharm. D., deserves special mention for his assistance.

Parents who were especially helpful include Betty Britt, Rick and Jayne Green, Anne Jacka, and Lenore Horowitz.

Mary Jones, Bonnie Obrig, and Virginia Arnone are the workers who converted our ideas to manuscript pages. Along with our editor, Elinor Neville, they merit special recognition for making this a book.

# Contents

# Preface

A CHILD'S HEALTH depends on parents' abilities to make sensible decisions. We believe that parents are often frustrated in their decision-making because of the lack of access to medical information that they are capable of understanding and using. Ideally, a good relationship with your child's physician should be a learning process in which you are encouraged to take responsibility for making decisions when your child becomes ill. In fact most childhood illness is managed by parents without a physician's help. However, parents must cope with considerable uncertainty before and even after they visit the doctor. In order to help you decide whether a symptom requires urgent medical attention, a visit to the physician today, a phone consultation, or home treatment, we collaborated in writing *Taking Care of Your Child*. This book is different. It focuses on providing you with information you need to decide whether your child truly requires a medication to improve and if so, how you should use the medicine and what you must know to ensure its safe and efficacious use.

Why do we need this book? Is this not what doctors and pharmacists tell us? The truth is that patients often leave the offices of physicians and pharmacists with considerable confusion and many unanswered questions. One study of patients leaving their doctors' offices revealed that over 50% made at least one error when describing what their physicians expected. This is not surprising, for recordings of the medical visits revealed that the doctors did not even discuss 20% of the medicines they prescribed. For 30% of these medications the doctors gave no information about the name or purpose of the drug. Of these patients, 90% were not told by their doctors how long to take the medicines, and less than 5% of the prescription bottles contained this information. Clearly, then, there is a need for both better communication between doctors and patients as well as information to make young patients and their parents better informed.

We believe that if parents are knowledgeable about medical decisions a true dialogue can take place with your physician about the best treatment for your child. Implicit in this statement is the assumption that a physician does not possess the "right" answer, but rather an educated opinion that considers such issues as trade-offs between the benefits and the risks of treatment, the manifestation of illness in your individual child, and the family and home environment. Because it is an opinion, we feel that there is room for discussion, negotiation and change, and that the parent should participate in this process.

It is probably clear by now that we do not feel that the physician's opinion is sacred and not to be challenged. This applies equally to the opinions expressed in this book. We have tried our best to present a balanced approach, and to label both fact and controversy; but in the end, much of what is said and recommended is the authors' interpretation of the facts. As such, we hope that you will not wave this book in your physician's face demanding to know why your child is not being treated according to the recommendations of Drs. Pantell and Bergman. We have intended that this book provide you with sufficient information to engage in a meaningful discussion with your physician about the best treatment for your child. It is not intended to, nor can it, provide the "right" answer for every problem.

## HOW TO USE THIS BOOK

This book is divided into four parts and can be used in a variety of ways. Part I discusses general issues involved in the presentation and treatment of illness in your child. This part is designed to convey the authors' philosophy on drugs and treatment, some tips on giving medicines to your child, and how to be an intelligent consumer of medicines. We feel that this section provides an important orientation and overview; it should be read in its entirety.

Part II describes the benefits and risks of using medications during pregnancy, labor and delivery, and the postnatal period. This section also describes the role of nutrition, nutritional supplements, and immunizations in preventing childhood illnesses.

Part III discusses medicine and treatments for specific conditions or situations. This part can be read in its entirety, or you can read just those chapters that apply to your child. Each of these chapters is divided into five sections: an introduction, which provides an overview of the problem; a rationale for treatment, which explains why we think that treatments and/or medicines are needed or not needed; a section on home treatments, which discusses what you can do without having to see your physician; a section on what additional treatment is available from your physician; and the fifth section, Is the Treatment Working?, intended to provide you with some guidelines for deciding whether or not a particular treatment is effective. In Parts II and III we use the generic names of medicines rather than brand names. In most cases the brand name is listed under the generic drug name in Part IV.

Part IV, Commonly Used Medicines, is a compendium of common medicines used in pediatrics. You can look up a particular medicine in this section and find the needed information without necessarily reading the accompanying chapters in Parts II and III. We recommend, however, that you read about the particular condition affecting your child, as well as read about the medicine, in order to get the best overall perspective on treating your child.

## WHAT THIS BOOK CANNOT DO FOR YOU

This book is not meant to be a guide to diagnosing illness in your child, or to help you decide when to take your child to the doctor. For this, we again recommend you read *Taking Care of Your Child* by Drs. Pantell, Fries, and Vickery. Our book is meant to assist you in making decisions about medicines and therapy *once a diagnosis has been made*.

This book will not provide you with the necessary information needed to treat your child by yourself. Although the sections on home treatment discuss what you can do without your physician, we also assume that a proper diagnosis has been made.

We hope that you are stimulated and educated by our book, and that this information will improve your skills and confidence in managing your children's illnesses and in teaching your children how to care for themselves.

*San Francisco, 1982*                                                      *D.A.B.*
*R.H.P.*

# Part I

# GENERAL ISSUES

# CHAPTER ONE

# Treating Your Child:
## *An Expanded View*

ILLNESS HAPPENS to everyone; it is part of growing up. As such it is an event when parents must exercise both judgment and caring in the treatment of their children. It is also an opportunity for parents to teach and children to learn how to manage an illness.

There is more to getting better than taking medicine. We feel that too much energy is expended by both physicians and patients in trying to eliminate each illness with medicine. Illness does not always require medication; it does require treatment. An "expanded treatment" is necessary for you to help your child recover from illness. This includes (1) the act of caring, (2) supportive home treatments including proper rest and nutrition, (3) over-the-counter preparations such as aspirin or nose drops, and (4) finally, medications that are not available over the counter but that require a doctor's prescription.

Before going any further you should take a moment to reflect on your relationship with your child's physician. Most good relationships will be characterized by a negotiation process between physician, parent, and child directed towards fostering maximum family participation in the medical care of the child. Your physician should encourage your ability to make independent decisions, and you should foster the same process in your child. Modeling is very important. If you frequently reach for a pill to solve problems, your child will quickly learn this behavior. If you need to take chronic

3

medications you must carefully explain what these medicines are for.

In order to understand our expanded approach to treatment it is important to describe what we mean by some commonly used terms.

*Symptom.* Pain is an example of a common symptom. However, there are many ways that pain can be perceived in our bodies and processed through our minds. Pain that comes from a heart problem may be experienced in the fingers. Some of us are more sensitive to pain than are others. Injury, infection, or emotional tension may produce pain that results in a headache. To further complicate matters, young children may often associate a bellyache with getting extra loving and attention. "I've got a bellyache" may mean, "I want you to read a story."

*Disease.* A disease has a set of properties that enables physicians to classify and label it. A particular disease, such as hepatitis, may cause neither symptom nor dysfunction; may cause symptoms alone, such as jaundice; or may cause severe symptoms accompanied by inability to function and even death. When a disease impairs function we experience illness.

*Illness.* This is an experience in which you feel that something is wrong. There may be illness without disease. Emotional stress may produce pain or fatigue sufficient to make you slow down. Sometimes experiencing illness is useful; it forces us to slow down and may even serve as a preventive measure to avoid disease.

To foster your child's ability to detect, manage, and cope with illness we should like to suggest the following procedure.

1. *When your child has a symptom.* Children's symptoms must be interpreted in the context of their usual behavior. Most often, you will know when your child is sick. In some fashion or another, illness often interferes with a child's usual pattern of behavior, and you may notice that your child is less energetic, more irritable, or has suddenly lost that usually ravenous appetite. What is oftentimes more perplexing is

when a child complains of a bellyache. Children are wonderful learners. A complaint of pain in the belly may be an imitation of what you said last night, or may in fact be a real symptom. Always model good behavior for children. Consider how you yourself deal with your symptoms, and encourage your children to truthfully report on their own. Even at a young age you can encourage children to describe what seems to hurt. Although the question "Are you sick?" is too abstract for a four-year-old to understand, most children that age will be able to point to parts of their bodies that are causing trouble.

2. *When your child is ill.* When younger children are ill you must take full responsibility for noticing, managing, and treating the illness. However, once the children reach the age of about six years, they can be given responsibilities for some of the decisions that occur during common illnesses. For example, they should share in the decisions about when they are ready to go back to school, and if they need to be in bed or up and around the house. They can let you know what foods they feel they can tolerate. Because children often wish to do things that exceed their abilities, as a parent you should make the final decision. However, you should reward sensible decision-making by praising a good decision, or foster better decision-making by challenging shaky judgments.

3. *When your child needs treatment.* Many treatments involve adhering to certain diets, rest, or limitation of activities. Again, starting at the age of about six years your child can be made to participate in the responsibility for these treatments. The best way you can encourage your child to do this is to suggest how important it is.

4. *When your child needs medication.* Younger children may not fully appreciate the precise ways in which medications fight infections or correct deficiencies. They nevertheless can learn, from an early age, that medication is important to feel better. Therefore, starting at the age of about six years, you can encourage your child to remind you about taking medications. Not until the age of about ten years

should children really have free access to the medication or be expected to perform this function on their own. However, between the ages of six and ten years, responsibility for taking medications can be shared so that the child is encouraged to ultimately take full responsibility for administration of medication during late childhood. Encouraging responsibility is important, but make sure that the children are acting responsibly. Children learn from the way their parents act. Always model good behavior by taking drugs only when needed. *Never* tell children that medicine is candy. It is obvious how this can lead to disastrous consequences. Also, do not use drugs as rewards or punishments.

# CHAPTER TWO

# Medications:
## *Principles of Therapy*

If you need to give your child a medication during an illness, there are some useful things to know about how medicines work. Whenever a medication is taken, the purpose is to improve the course of an illness, to maintain certain bodily functions, or to prevent certain events from occurring. For every drug your child takes there should be a targeted outcome. There are many categories of outcomes effected by medicine. The following are some illustrative examples.

| | **Targeted Outcome** | **Medication** |
|---|---|---|
| SYMPTOM RELIEF | *Reduce fever* | Acetaminophen, aspirin |
| | *Reduce sneezing* | Chlorpheniramine maleate |
| | *Reduce cough in pneumonia* | Dextromethorphan hydrobromide |
| DISEASE TREATMENT | *Eradicate bacteria in pneumococcal pneumonia* | Penicillin |
| | *Open airways in asthma* | Theophylline Epinephrine |
| DISEASE PREVENTION | *Asthma* | Cromolyn |
| | *Major motor seizure* | Phenobarbital |

The ability of a medication to be effective in accomplishing its task depends on a number of factors. First, you or your physician must make an accurate diagnosis. Second, a medication known to be effective for a targeted outcome must be chosen. This is usually the most difficult task. Although all new drugs must scientifically be proved effective before marketing, many older drugs were released before this law took effect. In addition, many drugs may be effective in combating one feature of a disease but ineffective in resolving another aspect of the same disease. For example, penicillin is effective in preventing some serious complications of a strep throat such as rheumatic fever. However, it is unable to prevent another unusual complication, kidney disease, and probably has little or no effect on the sore throat or fever accompanying the infection. Often your physician will make an accurate diagnosis but will prescribe a medicine based on his best, though not certain, estimate of the underlying cause. For example, in your community, your physician may prescribe ampicillin for an earache knowing that this agent will work to eliminate 90% of the types of bacteria responsible for this infection. No available antibiotic is effective all the time, and ampicillin will be ineffective in about 10% of these cases. This means that sometimes a second antibiotic will be necessary. Consequently, it is important to contact your physician if your child continues to appear ill after a medication has been started and taken properly by your child.

It is easy to be tricked into believing that medicine is effective when it has no effect at all. Most acute illness resolves spontaneously in a few days. Taking some penicillin tonight and feeling better tomorrow does not necessarily mean that the penicillin was responsible. You might have felt just as good without any medication. Do not run your own medication experiments on your children or yourself!

A medicine's effectiveness also depends on when in the course of an illness it is given. Penicillin can prevent rheumatic fever quite well in the first week following a strep throat, but its ability to stop this complication declines quickly thereafter.

Determining the right dosage is also important. Correct dosing depends upon many factors including your child's age and weight. Certain foods and drugs can interfere with a drug's absorption, as can diarrhea or vomiting. Other drugs may enhance a drug's absorption. Therefore, it is always important to check with your physician, pharmacist, or this book about drug interactions. Children with chronic kidney or liver disease are unable to eliminate all medicines efficiently. To achieve a similar drug level in these children usually requires a lower dosage of medicine than a healthy child requires.

Once the proper medication and dosage have been determined in order to achieve a targeted outcome, the real work begins. Medicine is ineffective on the shelf. It must get into your child to work. Because this is so important we have devoted the next chapter to a discussion of procedures that we believe will be helpful in medicating your child.

But before we move on to this practical advice, there are two more important principles to understand. Many parents worry about their children becoming "resistant" to the medication. This is actually known as developing a *tolerance* to the medication. In fact, this happens for only a few medications used in children. It occurs with narcotics, which include codeine, an analgesic pain reliever and cough suppressant. It also occurs with barbiturates, such as phenobarbital. This is actually beneficial to children, who develop a tolerance to phenobarbital's ability to make them drowsy while they remain susceptible to its property of preventing seizures. Most medications, including antibiotics, do not exhibit tolerance in children.

Finally, it is important to appreciate the power of the placebo effect. Through the years physicians have learned that patients often feel better after being given a pill, even when this pill has no active medicinal ingredients. Although this is seldom done in practice, it is part of most scientific studies done to determine the effectiveness of a new drug. In these studies, one group of patients will receive the drug while another group will receive a placebo that looks exactly like the new drug. Some remarkable things have been discovered about the power of placebos from these countless studies. In general, most placebos will achieve a targeted outcome in 30% of patients. If a placebo can reduce headache in nearly one-third of patients, does this mean that these patients did not truly have headaches? Not at all. Symptom relief is always a complex interaction that involves the pharmacologic properties of a drug, your belief in the clinical ability of your physician, and the susceptibility of your problem to medication relief. Hence, the placebo effect is very real. It is also a double-edged sword. We have heard patients attribute benefits to certain drugs that are not characteristic of these drugs' pharmacologic properties. However, the placebo effect is often beneficial. If you and your child believe in your physician's judgments and recommendations for medication, your child is already on the road to recovery thanks in part to the placebo effect. This underscores our belief in all patients having a relationship with their health care provider characterized by mutual respect, open lines of communication, and confidence in clinical competence.

# CHAPTER THREE

# Giving Medicine:
## *How to Remember*

PERHAPS THE GREATEST reason for treatment failures in children is the failure of the child to receive the medicine properly or to receive the medicine at all. The magnitude of this problem is considerable. Studies have shown that anywhere between 20% and 80% of children will not receive their medications or treatments properly. Why is there such a high failure rate in complying with medical treatments? The initial response on the part of many physicians is to accuse the parent of being careless and irresponsible. This response is unfortunate and leads to feelings of guilt on the part of the parents and a self-righteous attitude on the part of physicians.

*Compliance,* or administering all the prescribed medication, should be viewed as a dynamic process stemming from your relationship with your physician. In other words, good compliance is as much the responsibility of your doctor as it is yours. If we consider compliance as taking the prescribed amount of medicine at proper intervals for the correct reason, it is apparent that there is much a physician can do to help you. For example, he or she can reduce the number of medicines and the frequency of the doses of most medicines to make the treatment plan easier to remember and follow. It is much more difficult to remember to take several medicines at different times of the day than it is to take one medicine two or three times a day. Your physician can again help by making sure that you understand the nature of your child's problem, the reason for the medications, when and how the medication works, and what are the possible side effects. Without this level of understanding, you may lose confidence in the accuracy of the diagnosis and your physician. This can significantly compromise your willingness to comply with the prescribed treatment.

How much confidence you have in your physician can make a real difference in your compliance with the treatment. Parents who have developed a warm supportive relationship with their physician are more likely to believe in the diagnosis and to comply with the treatment regimen. The amount of stress in your life can also be influential. Families experiencing considerable stress (illness in a family can cause considerable stress) may have a difficult time harnessing the energy necessary to comply with the prescribed treatment.

From this discussion, it is apparent that good compliance demands a strong cooperative effort on the part of both you and your physician. What can you as a parent do to encourage good compliance in your family? First, make sure you fully understand your child's diagnosis and the reason for the medication. Ask questions! Do not feel pushy or stupid if you do not understand what your physician has told you. It is his or her responsibility to make sure that you understand what is wrong with your child. Remember, incomplete understanding of your child's diagnosis or treatment can affect your ability to administer medical treatment.

Be sure that your physician explains to you (1) how the prescribed medicine works; (2) how long it will take to work; (3) how you know if it is working; (4) what side effects it may have; and (5) what to do if any of these side effects occurs. Complete understanding of the medicine involved in your child's treatment will help you recognize both a medicine's potentials and its limitations.

Help your physician adapt the medicine regimen to your daily activities. For example, let your physician know that you will be at work or your child will be at school when the medicine is scheduled to be given, and that another time would be more convenient. Be sure that you have the simplest medical regimen possible. Even though you will not always have a choice in this matter, frequently your physician can prescribe another medicine that for a few extra dollars can be given less frequently without the need of additional medications.

At home, simple reminders can assist you in remembering to give medicines during a busy day. A picture of a clock with arrows drawn pointing at the times the medicine is to be given can be pasted on a frequently used appliance such as the refrigerator. This may be helpful in jogging your memory. Having the medicine packaged in a calendar pack or marking X's on a calendar may help you remember whether you have given the medicine that day.

There are tricks in administering medicines to children that can make compliance easier. For infants less than six months of age, the natural tendency is for the tongue to push out when it comes in contact with medicine. This makes giving medicine with a small spoon next to impossible. To circumvent this problem, use a syringe or a calibrated eyedropper to place the medicine in the pouch of the cheek toward the back, where it cannot be pushed out by the tongue. This technique is also a much easier and more accurate way to measure out the precise amount of medication necessary to give an infant. Although a teaspoon is supposed to hold 5 ml of medicine, the amount actually held can vary from 2 ml to 7 ml depending on the type of teaspoon you use.

For toddlers, the major problems in administering medicines are ones of taste and consistency. Parents have used numerous methods to disguise medicines that their children dislike having to take. Some of the more successful methods have included hiding the medicine in a highly liked food such as ice cream, freezing the medicine into popsicles, or following the administration of the medicine with a pleasant-tasting food to disguise the taste. Remember, it may be easier for some children to swallow a ground-up tablet in ice cream than it is to swallow a supposedly good-tasting liquid. (Taste the medicine yourself so you have some idea of what your child is confronting.) Whatever system you use to administer your medicine, inform your physician as to what you are doing. It may be that such a technique will alter the effectiveness of the medication.

Ultimately, every parent will participate in a knock-down, drag-out fight with their toddler or preschool-aged child over taking medicine. The child in this situation, with his or her ability to spit, vomit, and clench teeth, will win in a showdown every time. In fact, the more intense the struggle the more the child will relish the fight. In these situations it pays to draw back for a few minutes, let the struggle diffuse itself, and try again. This method may provide the toddler with enough sense of control that he or she will acquiesce to taking the medicine the next time around. The truly recalcitrant child is a difficult problem that should be discussed with your physician, who may be able to suggest an easier way to deliver the medicine (e.g., by syringe), or other approaches to giving that medication.

Enlist your child's help in remembering to take medicines. Provide him or her with encouragement and rewards for taking even a small part of the responsibility for taking medicine. This will also help your child feel that taking medicine is something that he or she can positively choose rather than something that is done whether he or she likes it or not. Last, it is important to remember that compliance with medical treatment is a difficult task for all of us; 100% compliance is neither a realistic nor an expected goal. You are only human and as such your physician should not expect you to be perfect in this respect. It is important, however, for you to let your physician know if you have not been fully able to comply with the treatment. To keep this lack of compliance a secret may lead your physician to draw the wrong conclusions about your child's illness and may cause more harm to your child than your not being able to fully follow the treatment plan. It is our hope that the information provided in this book will increase your understanding about what is being done for your child, and why it is being done, and will aid you in the difficult job of compliance.

# CHAPTER FOUR

# A Consumer's Guide to Buying Medicine

IN 1982 Americans will spend over $10 billion buying prescription drugs, and billions more on over-the-counter medications. There are estimated to be over one-quarter million medicinal products available on the shelves of pharmacies, supermarkets, and gas stations. The drug industry continues to maintain its position as one of the most profitable manufacturing industries in this country. Most medical journals have as much advertising as medical reporting contained in them. For example, of the twenty-eight largest circulating medical journals, twenty-five are distributed free because of drug industry advertising. Parents are also bombarded with drug advertising. One out of every eight television commercials is an advertisement for an over-the-counter medication. All these facts point to the importance of being a wise consumer. This care will potentially protect both your child and your pocketbook.

Several questions come to mind before a consumer can decide about the wisdom of purchasing a medicine. Is it safe? Is it effective? What is the price? Will the benefits of taking the medicine outweigh the costs? You must become actively involved in all these questions because, surprising as it seems, the products on your shelves are not guaranteed to be either safe or effective.

## IS IT SAFE?

It was not until 1938 that the U.S. Congress modified the

15

federal Pure Food and Drug Act of 1906 to require that drugs be safe before they can be marketed. Safety is a relative concept. No medication is 100% safe. Almost all drugs have the capacity to cause serious adverse reactions in an occasional individual. Although the risk may be as small as 1 in 100,000, this is little consolation if it is your child who has this serious reaction. When medications are released they have gone through a series of trials intended to determine their relative safety. However, by the time most drugs reach phase 4 trials, in which they have conditionally been approved, only several hundred patients may have taken the drug for over six months; usually several thousand will have been given the medication. As a result, infrequent reactions (less than 1 in 1,000) may not be detected before more extensive usage has occurred. In other words, it may not be a good idea to be the first to try a new drug. Although drugs since 1938 have had to pass a safety test, and although products marketed before 1938 are removed if they are considered unsafe, ·there may still be products available with a questionable safety record.

Almost all drugs in large doses are fatal. Some drugs are potentially lethal if only a few times the therapeutic dose is given; others have a much wider margin of safety. Be particularly cautious with psycho-active drugs, drugs that influence the central nervous system, such as sedatives, seizure medications, or heart preparations.

## IS IT EFFECTIVE?

In 1962 the Food and Drug Administration was charged with ensuring that all newly marketed drugs are effective as well as safe. The efficacy requirement was made retroactive to all drugs released after 1938, but exempts medications marketed before then. Many of these older drugs are still available.

Following a 1966 report in which an FDA-commissioned study determined that 75% of 400 common over-the-counter drugs were found to be less than effective for some or most of their claims, the FDA embarked on a series of steps to review available over-the-counter products. However, it will still be a number of years before you can purchase medications with the knowledge that they are both safe and effective.

The Food and Drug Administration limits its involvement in efficacy to restricting the claims a drug company can make in both its advertising and the package insert. The package insert is developed by both the drug company and the FDA and lists, among other information, approved indications for use of a drug. However, because the FDA has no jurisdiction in defining the limits of medical practice, physicians can prescribe approved drugs for nonapproved indications. In some cases their judgments are based on recently published scientific trials; other times they may be using a medicine erroneously or even for situations in which the drug is neither effective nor safe. Such was the case with diethylstilbestrol, a drug that is useful for a number of conditions but that is documented to cause vaginal cancer in the daughters of women who use the drug during pregnancy. Some physicians continued prescribing this drug to pregnant women years after the scientific literature and the FDA declared it unsafe during pregnancy. For reasons such as this, many consumer groups advocate that the package insert be given to all patients; others fear the the package insert's listing of precautions, contra-indications, warnings, and adverse reactions might unnecessarily frighten patients. Currently the best guarantee of your receiving effectual medication is having a competent physician who will discuss the role of any medication in the management of your child's illness. We have also addressed efficacy in the description of each drug in Part III.

## WHAT IS THE PRICE? WILL THE BENEFITS OUTWEIGH COSTS?

It is appropriate to be concerned with the price of drugs. In recent years, drugs have accounted for about one-tenth of our nation's medical bills. There are a number of steps that you can take to minimize the amount you spend on medications. First, always ask yourself and your doctor if the medication is really necessary. Most symptoms of common problems will disappear shortly if left alone. Is it really necessary for your child to take several medications for that runny nose when a few tissues might do as well? The "cost" of a medication includes the actual price of the medicine, the price of your time and gasoline expended to get to the pharmacy, as well as the price of managing any adverse or allergic side effects of the drug. Sometimes symptoms are sufficiently distressing to merit this cost of a drug; often they are not that severe. You must always consider whether the benefits of a medication outweigh its costs in terms of both money expended and potential side effects risked.

Second, compare prices. Many surveys have revealed that the price of a medicine can vary as much as ten-fold in a community. Typically, there will be a two- to three-fold variation in cost; a medicine priced at five dollars in one pharmacy may cost ten to fifteen dollars in another pharmacy. Some pharmacies post prices, most do not, but all should be willing to quote you a price over the phone. Pharmacies use a variety of methods to set prices. Charging an additional fee to their cost for the medicine, attaching a fixed mark-up, or a combination of these two procedures are the most commonly employed systems. Getting a low price on one medicine does not necessarily mean that all medicines will be the least expensive in a particular pharmacy. Although some pharmacies are uniformly less costly on prescription prices, it is important to remember the advice given in Chapter 5, Choosing Your Pharmacy. Saving a few cents in a pharmacy that keeps you waiting one-half hour and that has no pharmacist available to answer your questions may not be a worthwhile saving.

Third, medicines are usually less expensive when bought in large quantities. While some medications deteriorate rapidly, many have a long shelf life. If your child is on a chronic medication, always ask your physician to prescribe enough to last several months. This is cheaper than having frequent prescription refills.

Fourth, ask for generic prescriptions when possible. A generic name is usually the same as the official name of the drug listed in the *United States Pharmacopoeia*. This differs from the proprietary or trademark name given by a drug manufacturer. Considerable controversy exists concerning proprietary versus generic prescribing. Several points should be kept in mind. A higher price does not necessarily guarantee quality. For most medications generic medications are equivalent to proprietary drugs. Although some proprietary manufacturers may correctly claim that one of their particular drugs is better absorbed than an equivalent generic drug, this difference may not be important. This is usually true with antibiotics, antihistamines, analgesics, and many other types of drugs. For some preparations, such as theophylline, drug availability is far more critical and there is a basis for using proprietary drugs. In this situation it is usually important, when a dose is being changed, to continue the same proprietary drug. Taking the same dosage while changing to another proprietary or generic form with different absorptive properties may cause an unwanted elevation or lowering of the blood level of the drug.

Fifth, do not use a prescription for a drug that can be purchased over the counter. Many drugs that were prescription drugs years ago are now available over the counter at cheaper prices. Sudafed is just one example. Make sure that a drug is not available on the shelf before handing your prescription to the pharmacist.

## SOURCES OF INFORMATION ABOUT DRUGS

In addition to your physician, pharmacist, and copy of this book, other helpful publications are available in libraries and bookstores.

### PHARMACOLOGY BOOKS

These books probably contain more than you would ever want to know about medication, but they can be understood if you did not have too painful an experience with college-level chemistry and biology courses. Goodman and Gilman's *The Pharmacological Basis of Therapeutics* (Macmillan, 1980) is a standard text.

*AMA Drug Evaluations* is probably the most informative clinical reference in discussing information on efficacy. It is preferable to the *Physicians' Desk Reference,* which is essentially a collection of the package insert information issued by the drug manufacturters after FDA approval.

## BOOKS GEARED TO CONSUMERS

*The Medicine Show* has been published every year or two since 1961 by the Editors of *Consumer Reports,* and is a good general guide (and best buy!) to health products for adults.

*The Physicians and Pharmacists' Guide to Your Medicines* (Ballantine, 1981) is a comprehensive guide to prescription medications for adults and children by a panel of physicians and pharmacists.

*The Pill Book* by Silverman and Simon (Bantam, 1979) contains an exhaustive list of medications and side effects.

*The People's Pharmacy* by Graedon (Avon, 1980) is a popular book also directed toward providing insight into many of the controversial areas of medications. It is primarily directed toward adults.

# CHAPTER FIVE

# Choosing Your Pharmacy

Dorris Denney, Registered Pharmacist*

FREQUENTLY HEALTH CARE problems are handled by an individual or family without a visit to a physician's office. Think about it. You or someone in your family has a sore throat and a fever, so you stop at the drug store to pick up some aspirin and, perhaps, a bottle of mouthwash. A cough has been keeping your child awake at night, and you need some cough syrup. You are planning a long automobile trip and want to take some motion sickness pills before leaving. A sunscreen is needed for that summer vacation at the seashore.

Where do you buy these items? Do you ask for advice at the time they are purchased? Or are they purchased in a location where no health professional is in sight, such as at a convenience or grocery store? In these days of one-stop shopping and bargain hunting, we tend to forget the vital role that your local pharmacist and pharmacy make (or could make) in your health care. One hears about the importance of having one doctor to handle your family's medical problems. It is just as important to have one pharmacy for your family's drug needs and medical supplies. Consequently, one should put as much thought into choosing a pharmacy as in the selection of other health care providers.

In 1980, Schering, an independent research organization, conducted a study throughout the United States in urban, suburban, and rural areas to learn what consumers think

*Registered Pharmacist, Community Health Clinic, Nampa, Idaho.

about the pharmacy as a place to learn about and purchase over-the-counter medications. The results of that study indicated that 44% of consumers ask their pharmacists for advice on minor health problems at least once during the year. In addition, the majority of visits to a physician's office result in the writing of a prescription that must be taken to a pharmacy to be filled.

With these thoughts in mind, think about the importance of having confidence in your choice of pharmacy and individual pharmacist who will assume responsibility for the product and accompanying medical advice you will receive for your drug therapy. How carefully do you choose that pharmacy? What criteria do you use—convenient location, least expensive, friendly personality of the pharmacist?

The pharmacy can be a small, independent practice, or it can be part of a chain and located within a grocery store or discount store. Federal and state regulations are similar and certain minimum standards must be maintained by all.

Do not hesitate to ask the pharmacist about the nature and extent of services. Now is the time to find out that service is not available on Sunday. Most pharmacists should be willing to discuss their services; abrupt responses now will probably reflect abrupt services later. Before going to a pharmacy, you might make several phone calls to check comparative prices on a prescription item that you have needed before. Beware of a price that is way out of line with the majority.

The differences come in the degree of services offered, and these can be placed in four major categories, according to Kenneth B. Roberts, who presented a paper to the Idaho State Pharmaceutical Association entitled "Marketing a Professional Pharmacy Practice" (Coeur d'Alene, Idaho, June 14, 1981). The order of priorities will differ for the individual consumer.

1. Physical Characteristics of the Pharmacy
   a. convenient location
   b. clean atmosphere

    c. competitive prices

    d. good selection of products

    e. procurement of out-of-stock items when requested

2. Employees (nonprofessional and professional)

    a. courteous, helpful, friendly

    b. informative

    c. accessible

    d. concerned

3. Convenience Services

    a. provides after-hours emergency services

    b. has delivery service

    c. accepts third-party or Medicaid payment prescriptions

    d. mails medications

    e. provides credit or accepts major bank credit cards

    f. supplies prescription expense records for insurance or income tax purposes

    g. stocks surgical appliances

    h. has fitting room for surgical appliances

    i. has private consulting area

    j. has waiting area

    k. provides poison antidote and prevention information

4. Professional Services

    a. maintains patient profiles. These are records of all medications received from that pharmacy and enable the pharmacist to detect potential drug interactions, allergies, or misuse of medications. If an individual is receiving medications from another pharmacy, it is important that this be known to both. (How much easier it would be if you went to only one pharmacy!) The profile may be kept for an individual or for the entire family on one card.

    b. explains drug usage, dosage, storage conditions. It is not enough to simply count the right number of tablets, label the vial correctly, and hand the finished prescription to the patient in a paper bag. Receipt of your medication is the last step in the medical process. Therapy is now in your hands, and the more knowledgeable you are about the medication received, the better chance you will have for a more favorable outcome of your illness.

c. detects possible adverse reactions and incompatibilities and informs your physician.

d. provides a clearly labeled prescription with instructions for administration and any special warnings needed such as to avoid alcohol, dairy products, sunlight, etc. Also, provides easy-open caps for those individuals who have trouble with child-proof containers.

e. available for consultation on proper selection of over-the-counter products. (Again, this is much easier to do when allergies, concurrent medications, and chronic disease conditions are known by your pharmacist—another reason for having one pharmacy.)

f. is available for talks on topics such as drug abuse, poison prevention, and proper use of medications.

g. provides information on the proper use of medical and surgical supplies.

h. maintains confidentiality of your medical and personal problems.

As mentioned previously, the order of priority of these criteria will vary from one individual to another, and they will vary as the needs of you and your family change. The availability of surgical appliances and delivery service may not be critical to a young family, but may be very important to an elderly patient.

The price of medication will always be an important factor, but the quality of pharmaceutical products and service should not be sacrificed. The amount of money saved on a prescription initially may, in the long run, not be a true savings if other pharmaceutical needs are not met.

# CHAPTER SIX

# What Should Be in the Medicine Cabinet?

THE MEDICINE CABINET is often a warehouse that stores a variety of products including bathroom cleansers, hair dyes, birth control pills, and treatments for pets. Invariably there are medications: some current, useful, and necessary; others dangerous souvenirs of long-forgotten encounters with illness and injury. A cabinet with the characteristics of a treasure chest invariably beckons to treasure hunters. Unfortunately, although curiosity is the driving force that stimulates children's learning, it is also the reason why many children wind up in emergency rooms and hospitals being treated for dangerous and often fatal ingestions of household products and medications.

Virtually all medicine is fatal if an overdose is taken. Even though we are horrified when we read the occasional headline of a young child accidentally shot due to carelessness with a gun, lack of caution with medicine is so commonplace in our overmedicated society that it appears to be considered acceptable. It was unfortunately unacceptable to the hundreds of children who died last year from overdoses and ingestions. A bottle of medicine in the hands of a toddler is ultimately little different from a loaded gun. If you have young children at home, now is the time to clean out your medicine cabinet.

The best way to keep it safe is to keep it simple. First, make sure that cabinets have latches or locks that are out of reach; children always seem to be resourceful enough to be able to get at the cabinet itself. Second, keep your own medications separate and secure. They are usually dispensed in dosages where only a few tablets can be harmful to small children. Third, throw out left-over medications prescribed for old illnesses now.

## EQUIPMENT

*Thermometer*   You should always take your child's temperature if you suspect illness or a fever. Thermometers come in basically two styles, oral or rectal. Rectal are usually easier to use on younger children, and better approximate the child's internal temperature. Oral thermometers are acceptable in older children but must remain in the mouth at least for three minutes for an accurate reading. Oral temperatures may be inaccurate because of the effect of hot or cold foods, mouth breathing, or smoking. Their readings are about one-half degree Fahrenheit less than rectal temperatures. Underarm thermometers are inconvenient. The electronic thermometers you may have seen in your physician's office are too expensive (over $300) for home use. Either Fahrenheit or centigrade thermometers are acceptable. A level of either 101° Fahrenheit or the centigrade equivalent of 38.3° is generally considered to be indicative of fever or febrile illness. When taking rectal temperatures, place your child stomach down and insert the thermometer only an inch or two. A lubricant such as petrolatum (Vaseline) or K-Y jelly on the thermometer can facilitate matters; a hand on a baby's bottom with another hand behind the knees will stabilize the situation. Two minutes is enough time for an accurate reading; the mercury should no longer be rising after this.

*Cloth Tape*   One-inch tape is handy for holding a clean piece of gauze to an area of skin that needs shielding from the outside environment and its hazards. It is also useful in emergencies for applying splints, and can be torn and placed to bring together the edges of cut skin. It can also be used to increase strength and stability in healing an ankle (a special situation for your doctor to demonstrate). One word of caution: never encircle an entire extremity with tape. This can block circulation, cause pain and swelling, or even decrease function of the limb. A red, white, blue, painful, or swollen hand, foot, finger, or toe is in danger and needs a loosening or removal of the bandage.

*Gauze* A few 2 in. by 2 in. and several 4 in. by 4 in. pads should take care of most situations requiring a skin covering.

*Bandages* These time-honored treatments for minor cuts, scratches, and abrasions have a major role as a child's "red badge of courage." Younger children often worry that their bodies will leak out through a puncture wound—no wonder that bandages seem important! This is a good time to encourage their decision-making by allowing children to determine whether or not the severity of the injury warrants an intervention. Ask children if they feel they need a Band-Aid. Will it help, or merely draw attention to their misfortune? Would they like to keep one in their pocket just in case it's needed later? This acknowledges their misery without giving the message that all trouble requires concrete treatment.

*Tweezers* These have a variety of uses and are the best bet for removing splinters.

*Vaporizer* A vaporizer delivers a spray of tiny water droplets that reach into a child's upper air passages. It can provide dramatic relief for croup, an illness characterized by breathing difficulty and a barking cough that sounds like a barking seal. Croup is a common problem of toddlers that often begins suddenly in the middle of the night. Even though the steam created by the bathroom shower can be used if no vaporizer is available, it lacks the convenience of a bedside vaporizer. Cold steam vaporizers are best because they lack the risk of scalding that accompanies hot steam.

## TRAVELING MEDICINE CABINET

WHEN TRAVELING WITH CHILDREN you can never be sure that a pharmacy or medical care will be readily available. It is helpful to carry a few medicines in a traveling kit, to hold you over until you can reach a pharmacy and/or physician. We recommend:

*Aspirin or Acetaminophen* These medicines can help relieve the pain of minor injuries, an earache, and some symptoms of a cold.

*Cold Medicines* A decongestant or decongestant anti-histamine combination can be useful if your child comes down with a cold.

*Antibiotics* If your child suffers from recurrent urinary tract infections or ear infections and you plan to be on a camping trip away from medical care, we suggest you bring the antibiotic recommended by your physician with you. Here the risk of treating an infection that has not been documented by your physician is outweighed by the benefit of not having your child suffer for hours or days until you can reach medical care.

Your doctor may recommend a vaporizer for other upper-air-passage irritations.

*Elastic Bandages* These are useful for support after injuries and for securing emergency splints.

## MEDICATION

There are only three basic medications that are required:

1. aspirin (page 256) for fever, pain, and inflammations,
2. acetaminophen (page 249) for fever and pain,

If you are planning a long trip and your child is on chronic antibiotics or other medicines, take along an additional prescription (this may not be valid out of state) in case you need refills.

*Airplane Medicines* Many parents shudder at the thought of a 6 hour plane trip with a toddler, and request sedation for their child. Whereas this is an understandable goal, it is difficult to achieve. First, your child may be so excited by the trip that standard doses of sedation will have no effect and higher doses may be undesirable. Second, many children have a paradoxical response to sedatives and may be hyperactive for the trip. Third, if sedation is effective, your child will most likely be wide awake by the time you arrive, although you may be exhausted and ready for bed. If in spite of these warnings you still feel sedation is important, most physicians suggest antihistamine. Remember to test out the effects of the antihistamine *before* the plane trip. As the plane descends, ears can plug up. We recommend nursing or bottle-feeding infants and giving older children sugarless gum to chew. If your child has a cold, decongestants, either oral or topical may be useful in avoiding ear pain during ascent or descent.

3. syrup of ipecac (page 287) to produce vomiting in children who have accidentally swallowed pills or other substances for which vomiting is a suggested treatment. It is also a good idea to keep a bottle of ipecac in your car's glove compartment. Children often ingest medicines at older relatives' homes; having ipecac on hand immediately can save valuable time.

*Other good items to have around include:*

**Sun Screen** Products with the ingredient PABA (p-amino

benzoic acid) effectively block out some of the sun's rays and can reduce the risk of sunburning.

*Hydrogen Peroxide*  Scrubbing with soap and water is the best way to clean a dirty wound. Hydrogen peroxide is also an effective cleanser, which may remove additional dirt through its foaming action. Caution! Do not use in strengths greater than 3%.

*Betadine*  This nonstinging iodine preparation is an effective but expensive cleanser. Iodine also can be harmful in excess quantities. Only rarely are expensive antibiotic ointments better than soap and water.

  *Optional items with occasional use in relieving symptoms include:*

*Nose Drops*  Never to be used for longer than three days, for the lining of the nose can become dependent on nose drops. The simplest form of nose drops can be made at home by dissolving a teaspoon of salt in an eight-ounce glass of water. You can purchase preparations over the counter that act by constricting the blood vessels and membranes of the nose. Short-acting preparations contain phenylephrine and are available commercially as Allerest, Contac, Coricidin, Neo-synephrine and Sinarest. Neo-synephrine is available in lower concentrations (¼%, ½%) for younger children. Longer acting preparations contain oxymetazoline (Afrin, Duration, and St. Joseph Decongestant for Children).

*Cough Suppressant*  A cough is usually produced by the reflex action of the breathing passages responding to an irritant. Most reflexes are protective and in this case may serve to clear the airways of excess fluids or debris. However, a cough that interferes with a child's sleeping or that severely impedes functioning should be treated. There are several effective cough suppressants, including codeine and dextromethorphan hydrobromide. Because of its safety, we recommend dextromethorphan for children (page 272).

*Antihistamines* Although these are valuable for children with allergic problems such as hay fever, we feel that this class of drugs is questionably effective in treating colds. Having some diphenhydramine hydrochloride (Benadryl) available may prove useful in controlling an allergic response to another medication or to an insect sting.

*Oral Decongestants* This class of compounds has come under increasing scrutiny. They act by constricting blood vessels in the nose that deliver chemical substances responsible for swelling the nasal lining and producing mucus. Unfortunately, other blood vessels constrict as well, which may be responsible for a mild, short-lived elevation of blood pressure. One question is whether this is a reasonable trade-off for temporary relief of a symptom that is primarily a nuisance. Decongestants have not been shown to be effective in preventing or treating ear infections, the most common complication of colds in children.

*Cooling Shake Lotions (Calamine)* These lotions are useful in diminishing the itching of a variety of rashes—from poison oak or ivy to chicken pox. Never apply these lotions over red, raw, weeping, or crusting areas of skin. If you are in doubt about using these lotions, contact your physician.

# CHAPTER SEVEN

# Accidental Poisoning

INGESTIONS, or accidental poisonings, comprise one of the most significant health problems affecting children today. It is expected that more than two million children will suffer from accidental poisoning in 1982 alone. Any time that you or your child is taking medicines, the risk of accidental poisoning exists. It is important for you as a parent to realize this risk and know how to combat it. Poison control centers have provided information for us with respect to the medicines and substances most frequently involved in accidental poisoning. The following list comprises those substances most frequently involved in accidental poisonings: plants, soaps, detergents-cleaners, aspirin, vitamins and minerals, cold medicines, perfumes and colognes, household disinfectants, deodorizers, household bleach, and psychoactive drugs. This next list is composed of those substances most likely to be involved in a poisoning in which the death of a child results: aspirin, psychotherapeutic drugs, petroleum products, solvents, and pesticides. Look at these lists, and stop for a moment. Ask yourself how accessible these medicines and substances are to your children. These medicines and substances should be located in a place that is inaccessible to your children.

What situations afford the highest risk for accidental poisoning in your children? To answer this question we have to consider the child, where the medicine or substance is in your home, how that medicine or substance is packaged, and the home environment. In identifying the child at greatest risk, we first have to consider his or her developmental abilities. For the infant 0–3 months of age, the greatest risk of accidental poisoning comes from the parent or caretaker accidentally giving too much medicine. It is important that you obtain from your physician or pharmacist a precise way of measuring out the exact amount of medication. The preferred methods are in calibrated eyedroppers or teaspoons, syringes, or calibrated medicine cups. Remember that the teaspoon that you find in your drawer can vary in the amount of medicine that it holds from 2 ml to 7 ml. Assuming that your teaspoon holds the prescribed 5 ml of medicine may lead to problems of underdosage or overdosage of your child. Changing the frequency of doses can sometimes cause accidental poisoning in the infant. If you miss one dose, do not give two doses the next time unless explicitly told to do this by your physician. The extra dose can cause the infant to receive too much medicine and it can lead to serious side effects.

The infant between four and seven months of age will explore the world around him or her by placing objects in the mouth. Although it is unlikely that your six-months-old will reach into your medicine cabinet and snatch your medications, an older brother or sister may give the baby medicine as part of an experiment or as part of their play. Because of this, your medicines must remain inaccessible even to your older children. The 7–12-month-old has the capability to crawl and creep and generally move about. He or she has also developed a fine pincer grasp with the hand and is able to place small objects in the mouth. For an infant of this age, anything at ground level is fair play. Medicines and poisonous substances kept under the sink or in lower drawers are all potential ingestants. The infant in this age group is particularly likely to ingest cleaning substances kept under the sink or in lower drawers. These substances, like your medicines, need to be kept in a place that is out of reach for infants and children. The child from one to two years old is not only completely mobile but can also use her or his motor skills for problem-solving. This means that your child is now able to place a chair under a cabinet, climb up on the chair, and reach into the cabinet. It may also mean that your toddler can figure out your child-proof locks or caps even if you have to smash your medicine bottle to open it. What this means is that keeping your medicine in a high place or assuming that it is safe because it has a safety cap is not adequate. Potentially lethal medicines and substances are most safely kept under lock and key.

How a medicine is packaged and where it is placed are important risk factors for potential poisoning. As frustrating as the safety caps are to you, they have been the greatest single advance in preventing childhood ingestions. All medicines and toxic substances have to be stored in containers that have safety caps. It is also important to remember that safety caps are *not* 100% foolproof. In many instances, an inquisitive toddler may be able to open a supposedly child-proof container. Because of this, your medicines have to be stored in a locked cabinet, preferably a cabinet that is locked with a key. Cabinets that have "child-proof cabinet locks" or cabinets that are "high up" are not 100% safe. Be careful to keep your medicines stored in their original containers, and make sure that the containers are properly labeled. Be particularly careful not to put medicines in containers that once contained edible substances, for your child will swiftly assume that the medicines are also edible. Do not let your child watch you take your medicine, for there is a great tendency to imitate your behavior. Also, do not tell your child that his or her medicine is "the same as candy" or "tastes like candy," for this will confuse him or her. Labels exist to place on containers (see illustration) that graphically communicate to your child the undesirability of ingesting the substance or medicine inside. Teach your child to recognize that this label means that something bad or poisonous is inside, and that the container should not be touched.

High-risk situations for poisoning also occur during times of stress or disorder. Moving days, new babysitters, a sick child, or family strife are all situations that predispose to ingestions and accidents. It is unfortunate that those times when it is most difficult to be vigilant with your children are also the times that they are at greatest risk. If you know that you are going to experience a stressful time such as a moving day, it may pay to enlist a babysitter or other caretaker to attend to your child while your mind is on other things.

What should you do if an ingestion occurs? First, you need to anticipate that accidental ingestions will occur, and you should be prepared. You should have the phone number of your physician and your regional Poison Control Center nearby (you can obtain this latter number from your physician or from your phone book). These phone numbers should also be available to your babysitters and to any older brothers and sisters. You should have syrup of ipecac available in your medicine cabinet to induce vomiting when your Poison Control Center or your physician indicates that this is necessary. For some poisonings, inducing vomiting can be harmful. However, you can always give ipecac if your child has swallowed excess *medication*. Syrup of ipecac is available at your pharmacy or through your physician. If an ingestion occurs, try to find out what the involved substance was (save the container—it has important information on the label); determine a rough estimate of how much of the substance was ingested; and estimate at what time this occurred. Quickly determine if your child is listless, lethargic, or in severe distress, and then call either your physician or Poison Control Center. You should discuss ahead of time with your physician whether he or she prefers for you to call the office or call the regional Poison Control Center to find out what first steps should be taken. Do not rely on home antidotes or universal antidotes. They in general are not effective. Do not give the syrup of ipecac until instructed to do so by the appropriate health professional. If you are instructed to give the syrup of ipecac (the dose for your child should be determined in advance and written on the bottle) give it with 8–10 ounces of water. Then jiggle your child on your knee to mix things up and be prepared for vomiting within 10–15 minutes. If your child has not vomited after 20 minutes, let your physician or the Poison Control Center know to see if the syrup of ipecac should be given again. If your child vomits, try to save the vomitus (it can be helpful in determining what and how much was ingested) and bring it with you to the doctor.

In closing, we would like to note that we as parents must take a broader responsibility in decreasing the number of childhood poisonings that occur each year. We as a society have become casual with medications. We frequently assume that an ailment should be safely and easily resolved, and we often seek out a medicine as our first and only form of treatment. These behaviors result in the accumulation in the household of a myriad of medicines that are frequently forgotten about until the next illness occurs, and may become inactive or harmful over time. After you have finished using the medicine, the remainder of that medicine should be discarded and not saved for the next illness.

# Part II

# KEEPING YOUR CHILD HEALTHY

# CHAPTER EIGHT

# Medications During Pregnancy

By Maureen Shannon, C.N.M., F.N.P.*

FOR THE MAJORITY of parents, concern about the safety of medications and how they may affect their children begins during the prenatal period. Developing embryos and fetuses are particularly susceptible to the harmful effects of drugs because of the rapid growth and differentiation of cells that is taking place during this time. A very effective and efficient system of checks and balances exists between the fetus and the mother that serves to facilitate normal fetal growth and to protect the fetus from harm. However, this system is by no means totally foolproof. Some undesirable substances, including drugs, can be transferred in a number of biochemical ways from the mother to the fetus, adversely affecting the fetus.

An example of such a situation occurred during the 1960s with the drug Thalidomide. This particular tranquilizer was eventually associated with the development of limb deformities in infants of mothers who took the drug during pregnancy. Thalidomide had been tested for possible adverse effects by doing experiments on animals. Although limb deformities were not noted in the offspring of the experimental animals, the effect on human fetuses was very different. This unfortunate episode alarmed and further awakened the medical community regarding the possible harmful effects associated with drug use during pregnancy. It also reminds both medi-

*Certified Nurse Midwife, Family Nurse Practitioner, Upper Army Street Health Center, San Francisco, California.

cal professionals and consumers that the response of experimental animals to certain drugs can be very different from the human response.

Despite better education of medical professionals and consumers, women still use an average of four to ten drugs during their pregnancies. Many of these drugs are over-the-counter (nonprescription) medications that some women feel are "safe" to use for several reasons: (1) the women have used them before without problems occurring; (2) these drugs can be purchased without a prescription so they may be regarded as being "less" dangerous than prescription drugs; or (3) these drugs are used only "occasionally" (e.g. to relieve uncomfortable symptoms of common problems such as a cold). Unfortunately, no drug can be considered entirely safe during pregnancy. Many "safe" drugs can be harmful to the embryo or fetus if these drugs are taken in large doses, are taken over a prolonged period of time, or are taken during a particularly crucial part of embryonic or fetal development. For example, aspirin should not be taken during the last trimester of pregnancy because it can cause jaundice and (rarely) bleeding problems in the newborn infant.

Nevertheless pregnant women can, and do, become ill. In order to successfully treat some of these illnesses the administration of medications may be necessary. In these situations the physician recommends treatment because the risk of harm to the mother or her infant from the disease outweighs the risk of drug therapy. The risk-versus-benefit issue is more often overlooked when pregnant women use over-the-counter medications or the more accepted "social" drugs of our society (e.g. caffeine, alcohol, and nicotine). These social drugs are also associated with harmful effects of which pregnant women should be aware. Heavy alcohol use (more than two alcoholic drinks a day) in some pregnant women has been correlated with birth defects, mental retardation, and small size in their infants. Pregnant women who smoke ten or more cigarettes a day are more likely to have babies who weigh less than babies born to nonsmoking mothers. The effects of maternal overuse of caffeine or marijuana on the fetus are not well documented; but it can be emphasized again that the abuse of any substance during pregnancy can subject the embryo or fetus to unnecessary harm.

Table 1 lists many common drugs (prescription and non-prescription) and their potential harmful effects on embryos and fetuses. It is because of these harmful effects that a woman considering the use of any drug during her pregnancy should consult with her physician about the specific drug and her particular problem or need for its use; and then weigh the risk versus the benefit from its use.

TABLE 1
PRENATAL DRUGS AND POSSIBLE EFFECTS ON FETUS

| Drug | Amount | Possible Effects |
|------|--------|------------------|
| ALCOHOL | *Chronic use* | Birth defects; fetal alcohol syndrome; growth retardation; hypoglycemia |
| AMPHETAMINES | | Birth defects |
| ASPIRIN | *During last 3 months of pregnancy* | Neonatal jaundice (yellow skin due to increased bilirubin in infant's system); increased chance of bleeding problems in newborn |
| ANTIHISTAMINES | *Chronic use* | Seizures during neonatal period |
| ANTIBIOTICS *Streptomycin* | *Therapeutic dose* | Hearing loss |
| *Sulfa* | *Therapeutic dose during last 3 months of pregnancy* | Jaundice |
| TETRACYLCINE | *Therapeutic dose* | Dark staining of teeth; malformed teeth; decreased bone growth |
| BARBITURATES | *Chronic use* | Withdrawal symptoms during neonatal period (e.g. irritability, seizures) |

TABLE 1 (CONTINUED)
PRENATAL DRUGS AND POSSIBLE EFFECTS ON FETUS

| Drug | Amount | Possible Effects |
|---|---|---|
| CAFFEINE | *Chronic heavy use* | *Growth retardation |
| DIURETICS | *Chronic use* | Salt and water imbalance and/or depletion |
| DILANTIN | *Chronic use* | Birth defects |
| ESTROGENS | *Therapeutic dose* | Vaginal cancer |
| MARIJUANA | *Chronic use* | Unknown |
| METRONIDAZOLE (FLAGYL) | | Mutations in bacteria; cancer in rats |
| NARCOTICS e.g. heroin, methadone | *Chronic use* | Growth retardation; withdrawal symptoms during neonatal period |
| NICOTINE | *10 or more cigarettes per day* | Lower birth weights (smaller babies) |
| PROGESTINS Progesterone | *Therapeutic dose* | Masculinization of daughter |
| TRANQUILIZERS e.g. Thorazine | *Therapeutic dose* | Problems with temperature regulation; decreased levels of alertness |
| VITAMIN C | *High doses* | Skin and intestinal problems in neonate |
| VITAMIN D | *High doses* | Heart valve problems |
| VITAMIN K | *High doses* | Jaundice; *bleeding problems in newborns |

*These findings have been suggested but not proven.

# CHAPTER NINE

# Drugs During Labor, Birth, and in the Nursery

By Maureen Shannon, C.N.M., F.N.P.

THE EFFECTS OF DRUGS on infants remains an issue as pregnancy comes to a close with the beginning of the mother's labor. Both parents and physicians are acutely aware of the vulnerability of the baby to any potentially harmful effect of a drug as the woman's labor progresses through to the actual birth of the infant.

In most normal labors and births, the main problem that may require medication for the mother is the symptom of pain. Today, more and more parents are attending childbirth classes prenatally to learn exercises and breathing techniques that will help the mother cope with the uncomfortable aspects of labor. This preparation can decrease or eliminate the woman's need for analgesics (pain medications) during this time. However, some women do need to use analgesics during labor, and information about the drugs that may be used should be made available to them during their prenatal visits. Again, the physician should clearly delineate the risks versus the benefits of each option and answer any questions that the parents may have regarding the medications.

There are two basic classes of pain medications that can be administered during a woman's labor—systemic analgesics and local analgesics. The systemic medications are drugs that can be given by injection (into a vein, muscle, or subcutaneous tissue) to the woman, and that then circulate through her blood vessels. Narcotics (e.g. morphine) or synthetic narcotics (e.g. Demerol) are the most familiar drugs in this class. These medications decrease a woman's sensation of pain within ten to twenty minutes after their administration. The effectiveness can last from one to three hours depending upon how much medicine is given and which method is used to administer it. Drugs given intravenously get into the body, reach a peak level of effectiveness, and are excreted faster than drugs given into muscles or subcutaneous tissues. Transfer of the drug from the mother to the fetus does occur, and, over time, the drug is excreted from the fetus's system as well as from the mother's system. A few important transient side effects can occur in the fetus when these drugs are used. After administration of the drug to the mother it has been noted that there can be a decrease in the fetus's heart rate. Generally, this effect resolves within a short period of time when the majority of the drug has been eliminated from the fetus's system. Another side effect is that of drowsiness, which can be observed in infants who are born with too much of the drug in their systems. The treatment for this effect depends upon the severity of the symptom. If the baby is minimally drowsy, then simply stimulating the infant after birth by stroking her or him may be enough. When infants are born with drowsiness so severe that it impairs their breathing, then more vigorous types of treatment are indicated, such as the administration of oxygen and/or drugs to reverse the effects of the narcotic. To avoid these situations, most physicians and nurses carefully time the administration of a drug given to a woman in labor so that it will not be in either her system or the infant's system when the birth occurs. In situations where the fetus is already showing signs of problems, narcotics are often not used so that the fetus will not be further stressed.

Local analgesics were once used quite frequently to eliminate the pain associated with labor. The most common one was a paracervical block, which was an injection of a "caine" drug (e.g. Lidocaine) into the woman's cervix. This procedure would decrease the sensation of pain in the woman's cervix during the first stage of labor (during cervical dilitation). Paracervical blocks are no longer in favor because in some instances there would be a significant decrease in the heart rate of the fetus after this procedure was done. A significant decrease in a fetus's heart rate is often indicative of excessive stress and associated with a decrease in oxygen to the fetus. For the most part, the decreases in fetal heart rates that occurred in relationship to paracervical blocks would be resolved within a short period of time. On occasion this side effect persisted for a prolonged period of time—sometimes resulting in more stress and problems in the newborn. Consequently this procedure is rarely done today to relieve a laboring woman's cervical discomfort.

A pudendal block is another type of local anesthesia that may be used when a woman experiences pain during the pushing stage of labor. This anesthesia also uses one of the "caine" drugs; but the medication is injected through the vaginal wall into the nerves that transmit pain sensation to the vagina (not cervix) and part of the rectum. Women who have this anesthetic can still feel contractions and push with them. However, the pain that occurs in the vaginal area when the baby is being pushed out is eliminated. Often this anesthetic is used when a physician must use forceps to help with a baby's birth. Because this anesthetic is most often used when a baby will be born within a short period of time, there is little chance of the "caine" drug entering the baby's circulation and adversely affecting her or him.

Some women have problems during pregnancy or labor that may require special treatment with specific medications. Oxytocin (Pitocin) is one such drug used to stimulate labor and/or strengthen the uterine muscle during labor. Magnesium sulfate is a drug used in women who have severe preeclampsia (toxemia) to prevent them from seizing. The physician's management of such complications always focuses on the welfare of both the mother and the fetus. The use of drugs in these situations is always viewed in terms of benefits versus risks to both patients. Nevertheless, informed consent by the parents is required; and if it is not an emergency situation, the physician should answer the parents' questions about the drugs that might be used.

## CESAREAN BIRTHS

Although the majority of labors and births are normal and progress without the need for medical intervention, there is still a 10–20% chance that a pregnant woman in this country will give birth by cesarean section. The reasons for this are numerous and include problems such as (1) cephalopelvic disproportion—the baby's head is larger than the mother's pelvis: (2) fetal distress—the baby may have a problem that requires her or his immediate birth; (3) breech—the baby is positioned in such a way that a vaginal birth may be harmful to her or him; (4) multiple babies—twins, triplets, etc; or (5) maternal illness—the mother may have a severe illness that would make labor and/or a vaginal birth too dangerous or difficult for her.

Until recently women undergoing a cesarean section were asleep for the surgery. In many communities today women are being offered the choice of being either awake or asleep for this surgery. These options pose questions about the various types of anesthesia they may have and the risks associated with each type for both the mother and the fetus.

There are two types of anesthesia for cesarean sections—a general anesthesia or a regional (spinal) anesthesia (see Table 2). General anesthesia is the type that puts the mother to sleep for the surgery. It often combines an intravenous medication (such as sodium pentathol) with an inhalant (such as nitrous oxide). It is often used in emergency situations because the anesthesia gets into the mother's system rapidly so that the surgery, and the baby's birth, can occur within a very short period of time. Usually the infant is born without any problems within five to ten minutes after the mother goes to sleep. Rarely, infants are born drowsy because some of the medication entered into their systems, too. In these instances the baby may be less alert or responsive immedi-

TABLE 2
MATERNAL DRUGS THAT MAY BE USED DURING LABOR AND
DELIVERY AND POSSIBLE ADVERSE EFFECTS ON FETUS AND NEWBORN

| Drug | Reason for Use | Possible Adverse Side Effects on Fetus and Newborn |
|------|----------------|---------------------------------------------------|
| GENERAL ANESTHESIA e.g., inhalation of medicines— nitrous oxide | *Often used as anesthesia for cesarian births; can be used for pain relief and relaxation during vaginal births* | Decreased fetal heart rate; decreased alertness, responsiveness; decreased respirations |
| MAGNESIUM SULFATE | *Moderate to severe pre-eclampsia (to prevent seizures in mother)* | Decreased muscle tone, alertness, responsiveness of newborn (unusual); urinary retention (rare) |
| NARCOTICS e.g., Demerol, Nisentil | *Maternal pain relief* | Decreased fetal heart rate (usually transient); drowsiness, decreased respirations at birth (if given too close to time of delivery) |
| OXYTOCIN (PITOCIN) | *To stimulate or enhance uterine contractions* | Increased chance of jaundice in newborn |
| PARACERVICAL BLOCK *using any of the "caine" drugs— e.g. Lidocaine* | *Maternal pain relief during labor* | Decreased fetal heart rate (often transient); convulsions (rare) |
| PUDENDAL BLOCK *(using one of the "caine" drugs)* | *Maternal pain relief during pushing stage and birth of baby* | None |
| REGIONAL ANESTHESIA e.g. "spinal" *epidural block, caudal block with various types of "caine" drugs used* | *Maternal pain relief during labor and vaginal birth; can be used for cesarean births for anesthesia* | Decrease in maternal blood pressure can occur. If sustained there can be a decrease in oxygen to fetus with a decrease in respiration and alertness, decrease in responsiveness |
| TRANQUILIZERS e.g., Vistaril | *To decrease maternal anxiety during labor* | Drowsiness, decreased responsiveness |

ately after birth, and, in some cases, for a short period of time thereafter.

When women want to be awake for a cesarean birth a regional anesthesia (e.g. epidural or "spinal") is used. This type of anesthesia can block sensations of pain from the abdominal area to the toes. Once the anesthesia takes effect the baby is usually born within five to ten minutes. In healthy women and fetuses this type of anesthesia is rarely associated with any harmful effects. The most dangerous situation occurs when a woman's blood pressure lowers because of the anesthetic. This causes a subsequent decrease in the amount of blood and oxygen that is available to the fetus. However, for the great majority of women who choose this method of anesthesia there are no adverse effects on their infants or themselves. The numbness that the mother experiences lasts for approximately six to eight hours and usually resolves without problems.

## MEDICATIONS IN THE NURSERY

The first few hours after birth are recognized as an important "getting acquainted" period for the parents and the infant (i.e. the "attachment" or "bonding" process). Today most physicians and nurses are aware of the significance of this process, and they try to be as unobtrusive as possible while they carry out some important duties to ensure the safety of the mother and the infant. One of the procedures that usually occurs within a short period of time after birth is the administration of medications to the newborn to prevent some specific complications from arising.

The instillation of medication into the newborn infant's eyes is generally accepted as a necessary routine procedure in hospitals. The reason for this procedure is to kill any gonorrhea bacteria that may have come in contact with the infant's eyes during the birthing process. Gonorrheal infection of the newborn's eyes can rapidly lead to blindness. In approximately 90% of women gonorrheal infection will not produce a symptom; and therefore a woman may unknowingly have the bacteria existing in her cervix. Even though most pregnant women have cervical cultures taken to screen for gonorrhea, this test is only 80–90% accurate when it reports a negative finding (meaning that no gonorrhea is present in the woman's cervix). This fact leaves a 10–20% possibility that a woman with gonorrhea in her cervix may have a false negative reading on the culture. Taking this a step further, it means that this woman can unknowingly expose her infant to gonorrheal infection of the eyes.

There are two medications that are commonly used to eliminate the possibility of this eye infection in the infant— silver nitrate drops or erythromycin ointment. When silver nitrate is used it is gently dropped into the infant's eyes and, after a few seconds, sterile water is used to gently rinse the medicine from the infant's eyes. There are a few harmless reactions to this drug that have been observed in infants and that often worry parents. The silver nitrate can cause a tannish-brown discoloration of the skin around the eyes, which rapidly fades within a few days. Also, most infants develop a whitish-yellow discharge from their eyes and some puffiness of the eyelids because the medicine causes some irritation of the eyes. However, these symptoms are not indicative of an infection, and they will subside within a few days.

The erythromycin ophthalmic ointment does not cause any skin discoloration; and generally there is very little eye discharge or eyelid puffiness associated with its use. Often it does cause a slight film or coating on the eye for a few hours after its administration. This film can blur the infant's eyesight, which some parents feel will interfere with the parent-infant bonding process. This problem can be solved to some degree by having nurses or physicians wait until one hour after birth before administering the medication so that parent-infant bonding can be facilitated by eye-to-eye contact during the first hour after birth.

The one other medication often routinely administered to newborns is vitamin K. This vitamin is essential for blood coagulation and is produced by a specific enzyme system in the body. Although infants are born with all their organs and body systems functioning, some of these systems are still slightly immature. One of these is the enzyme that helps synthesize vitamin K. In order to avoid any problems with the infant's blood-clotting ability, it is recommended that a small dose of vitamin K be given by an injection into the infant's thigh muscle. This is especially important if a male infant is going to be circumcised. In rare instances, and usually in doses well above the required amount for newborns, this vitamin is associated with an increase in jaundice in the newborn.

In some hospitals parents who do not want their infant to receive any of the above routine medications can sign a "waiver" for omission of these procedures. This waiver is a legal document that usually states that the parents are refusing a specific medication or procedure for their infant after they have had the risks of such a refusal explained to them by their physician. When the waiver is signed it releases the physician and the hospital of legal responsibility for any consequences in the infant that result because of the parents' refusal of the administration of the medication.

# CHAPTER TEN

# Breast-Feeding

By Maureen Shannon, C.N.M., F.N.P.

RENEWED INTEREST in breast-feeding has stimulated an increased desire by, and a need for, mothers to know about the transmission of drugs through breastmilk to their infants. Technically, any drug taken by a mother can be found in very small amounts in her breastmilk. Consequently, the need for a mother to take a particular drug should outweigh the possible adverse effects that this drug may have on her infant, especially if it is excreted in large amounts in her milk.

How much of a drug is excreted in a mother's breastmilk and how much of a chance that this drug may be harmful to her infant are dependent upon the interaction of several factors. One of the factors that immediately comes to mind is the dose of the drug. Generally, a large dose of a drug will have more of a chance to get to the infant through the breastmilk than will a very small dose. Nevertheless, even small doses of drugs can pass through to the infant in significant amounts if the drug is taken often enough (e.g. every two hours); and/or if it is taken in small doses over a prolonged period of time (for several days or weeks). Some drugs have more of a tendency to bind to substances in the human body that have a large fat or protein component, or prefer more of an acidic rather than an alkaline environment (or vice versa). Breastmilk is more of an alkaline substance, and is higher in carbohydrate and fat content than it is in protein. How a particular drug will be transmitted through

TABLE 3
DRUGS IN BREASTMILK

| Drug | Amount | Possible Adverse Effect on Infant |
|---|---|---|
| ALCOHOL | *Chronic use* | Drowsiness, vomiting |
| ANTIBIOTICS | | |
| penicillin | *Therapeutic dose* | Occasional diarrhea |
| *tetracycline | *Therapeutic dose* | Tooth discoloration |
| *chloramphenicol | *Therapeutic dose* | Low blood count |
| ANTIHISTAMINES | *Chronic use* | Inhibition of lactation |
| ASPIRIN | *Chronic use* | Decreased blood clotting |
| BARBITURATES | *Occasional use* | None |
| | *Chronic use* | Drowsiness/withdrawal symptoms (irritability, seizures); decreased sucking reflex |
| CAFFEINE | *Chronic use (heavy)* | Jitteriness |
| DECONGESTANTS | *Long-term use* | Irritability, excessive crying |
| *DILANTIN | *Therapeutic dose* | Vomiting; low blood count |
| HORMONES | *Therapeutic dose* | Inhibit milk production; breast engorgement |
| LAXATIVES | *Therapeutic dose* | None |
| | *Chronic use or abuse* | Diarrhea |

*Contraindicated in breast-feeding women.

breastmilk depends upon its affinity for this type of environment. Often the drug prefers the biochemical composition of the mother's tissue and bloodstream to that of breastmilk, so there is less movement of the drug from the mother's sytem into her breastmilk and to her infant.

The timing of taking a drug in relationship to the time the infant will probably be breast-feeding is another factor. Often a drug can be taken so that there will be much less of it in the mother's system (and in her breastmilk) when the infant is going to nurse. How often an infant needs to nurse correlates with this, too. Often a mother can take a medication

TABLE 3 (CONTINUED)
DRUGS IN BREASTMILK

| Drug | Amount | Possible Adverse Effect on Infant |
|------|--------|-----------------------------------|
| MARIJUANA | Chronic use | Drowsiness |
| *METRONIDAZOLE (FLAGYL) | Therapeutic dose | Cancer in rats |
| NARCOTICS | Occasional therapeutic dose | Drowsiness; occasional constipation |
| *heroin | Chronic use | Addiction/withdrawal symptoms |
| *methadone | Chronic use | Addiction/withdrawal symptoms |
| NICOTINE | Chronic use | Inhibition of lactation; diarrhea, vomiting, restlessness |
| *RADIOACTIVE DRUGS | Excessive radiation exposure | Long-term effects of this unknown |
| RESERPINE | Therapeutic dose | Nasal stuffiness |
| SEDATIVES | Therapeutic dose | Drowsiness |
| THYROID DRUGS | Therapeutic dose | Goiter |
| TRANQUILIZERS e.g. Valium | Therapeutic dose | Drowsiness |

*Contraindicated in breast-feeding women.

after her infant has nursed and be fairly certain that very little will be in her breastmilk if the infant will not be nursing again for another four to six hours (e.g. during the night). Difficulty can occur when a woman needs to take a medication four times a day or every six hours, and her infant needs or wants to nurse every two to three hours. In situations like this the physician should consider using another type of drug that needs to be taken only twice a day instead of every four hours. Another option the mother has is to offer her infant a bottle of either her breastmilk (which has been expressed and saved from previous nursing periods) or a formula for one or two feedings when the medication she is taking may still be excreted in large amounts in her breastmilk. Some drugs should not be taken by women who are breastfeeding, and these drugs have been listed in Table 3. In rare situations when she must take a medication that is known to be harmful if transmitted to her infant through her breastmilk, a mother can formula feed her infant for the period of time she is on the medication. During this time she should continue to express her breastmilk (either manually or by using a breast pump) so that she will continue to produce it, and resume nursing her infant as soon as the drug is out of her system (this may be a number of days depending upon the drug).

When the topic of drugs in a woman's breastmilk is presented it is often the prescription drug that immediately comes to mind. However, over-the-counter drugs and "social" drugs (caffeine, nicotine, alcohol) also pass through breastmilk to infants, and can cause adverse side effects in some of these infants. For example, the excessive intake of caffeine (coffee and colas) by a mother can cause in her infant symptoms of jitteriness that will usually subside with the elimination of caffeine in her diet. Consequently the suggestions made to women about drug use of any type during pregnancy should also apply to women who are breast-feeding their infants (e.g. only two cups of coffee or cola a day; no more than two alcoholic drinks a day; and no smoking).

Maternal exposure to environmental pollutants and the effect of these substances on a woman's breastmilk is another area of concern. Unfortunately, the amount of information available regarding this subject is limited. The information that is available about the effects of certain toxic substances (e.g. DDT, PCB, THC) on breastmilk of women exposed to them has not revealed any substantive evidence of problems in their infants primarily because the amount of the substances measured in the breastmilk was very small. However, we are still unsure of the effect on infants exposed to larger doses of these substances or even to small doses of them over a long period of time. Whenever you are unsure

## WHAT'S A PARENT TO DO?

1. Read and/or ask questions of your physician for information and clarification about important issues in your care (e.g. medications, procedures).

2. Make sure that your physician or dentist knows that you are possibly pregnant, pregnant, or breast-feeding.

3. Remember that some maternal illnesses must be treated with medications (e.g. bladder infections) so discuss with your physician the benefits versus risks to you and to your baby of these medications.

4. If you are breast-feeding and you need to take medications, figure out with the physician the best time to take them so that these medications will have the least possible chance to get through your milk to the baby.

5. Be careful about the use of over-the-counter drugs and "social" drugs; these can have harmful effects on your baby also.

6. In rare instances a mother must stop breast-feeding because she is in need of a medication that may be harmful to her baby. Don't worry! Bottle-feed your baby with a formula and pump your breasts, discarding the milk. Resume breast-feeding your infant as soon as possible (and safe) after you have finished the medication. The baby may need a little time and coaching to nurse as well as she or he did before you had to stop—but the baby (and you) can do it!

of the safety of a substance you may be exposed to (e.g. environmental spraying, household cleaners, industrial chemicals) you should contact your physician and attempt to reduce or eliminate further contact with that substance until you have more information regarding its safety.

# CHAPTER ELEVEN

# Infant Formulas

IT IS BEYOND THE SCOPE of Part II to discuss the relative merits of breast- and formula-feeding as well as the specific techniques. These subjects have been covered in *Taking Care of Your Child* as well as in *Nursing Your Baby* by Karen Pryor (New York: Pocket Books, 1975). The American Academy of Pediatrics also has a helpful manual available from your pediatrician. Although we are strong advocates of breast-feeding, this method is not always possible and it is important for mothers to realize that both breast-feeding and bottle-feeding supply sound nutrition as well as intimacy to the baby. Remember, your baby will be happy when you are happy, so choose the method that will create the least stress in your life.

Both breastmilk and infant formulas (Similac, Enfamil, SMA) are nutritionally complete in their ability to provide sufficient calories to meet an infant's nutritional requirements for the energy needed to grow and be active. The American Academy of Pediatrics Committee on Nutrition suggests that for breast-fed infants, iron supplementation should begin at approximately the fourth month of age. It has also been recommended that solid foods need not be introduced until the sixth month of life, at which time iron-fortified rice cereal is generally begun. Make sure that the cereal package says *iron-fortified*. Some cereals, such as Pablum, do not have readily available iron. By seven months of age, fruits and then vegetables should be added singly on a weekly basis, culminating in the addition of meats by the end of the first year of life. Some physicians feel that the iron absorption from breastmilk is sufficient to obviate the need for supplemental iron in most children. However, some children may benefit from the iron supplementation recommended by the Committee on Nutrition. In addition, it is recommended that breast-fed infants should receive a vitamin D supplement if they live in a geographic area without much sunshine. Fluoride should also be given if it is absent from the local water supply.

Formula-fed infants should receive iron-fortified formula for the first six months of life. Vitamin D is present in the formula. Fluoride supplementation is similar to that for breastfed children. When iron-fortified cereals are added by six months of age, it is no longer necessary to feed the iron-fortified formula. Foods can be introduced in the same fashion as in breastfed infants. Iron absorption is increased by orange juice or by other products containing vitamin C.

It is important to avoid cow's milk in the first half year of life, including whole cow's milk, skim milk, and 2% fat milk. Cow's milk has the potential for increasing the risk of allergic problems in susceptible children, and it is notoriously low in iron, vitamin C, and copper. Skim milk is often begun in order to slim down a chubby baby. However, skim milk does not provide adequate calories; in addition it supplies an excess of sodium and protein.

Feeding a child breastmilk does not necessarily provide a guarantee against all the allergic and other problems of infancy. Mothers drinking large amounts of cow's milk have produced cow's milk allergy in their breast-fed babies. In addition, most drugs and chemicals that are ingested by mothers are passed on to babies in breastmilk. This includes caffeine, nicotine, alcohol, and the long list of drugs discussed in Table 3. However, it is extremely rare for mothers to have to discontinue breast-feeding because of problem symptoms in a baby. A careful dietary evaluation will most often identify a problem in your diet that may be causing a problem in your baby.

A word of caution. Virtually every symptom known has

been attributed to a child's being on the "wrong" formula. Children experience episodes of crying, fussiness, diarrhea, and spitting up for many reasons ranging from temperament to infection. It is important not to switch formula every time your child has a two-hour crying spell or a loose bowel movement. A very small number of children will, however, experience gastrointestinal allergy caused by the formula, or an allergic response elsewhere in the body triggered by the formula (eczema, asthma, allergic rhinitis). Other children may not be experiencing a true allergy but may be unable to digest a component of the formula (most often the milk sugar known as lactose), and consequently suffer from chronic diarrhea and abdominal distention. For children who are gaining weight poorly, who have chronic diarrhea, or who have problems with asthma or eczema the infant formula may be responsible. Although switching to soy formula is often the first and most rational approach, it is not always successful, for some children who are allergic to milk protein are also allergic to soy protein. Nonetheless, the switch to soy usually is the first step.

The following formulas have as their protein source soy instead of modified cow's milk: Isomil, Mulsoy, Neomulsoy, Nursoy, and Prosobee. They are all acceptable substitutes for known cow's milk allergy. Other specially treated formulas that can be used for cow's milk allergy include Nutramagen, Progestamil, and Vivonex. None of the above has lactose as its basic source of carbohydrate, and all are therefore useful for infants who are unable to digest lactose.

Other special formulas are available for children with diagnosed digestive problems. Portagen is used in children who have difficulty absorbing fat. Probana is a formula high in protein and low in fat that is also used for children with difficulties absorbing fat. Similac also makes a high-calorie formula, known as Similac 24, that is often prescribed for low-birthweight infants. There is also an Enfamil 24. Similac also has a product known as 60/40 for infants requiring low-salt diets or for those who have problems with calcium metabolism.

Pedialyte and Lytren are not true formulas in the sense

that they provide no protein or fat. They supply only dextrose, a sugar, as well as certain other elements, and they are most often prescribed during episodes of diarrhea.

# CHAPTER TWELVE

# Vitamins and Minerals

VITAMINS AND MINERALS are essential for your child's growth and health. Food is the best source of these nutrients. Healthy children, consuming an adequate, well-balanced diet, will not benefit from additional vitamins. Why then is the use of vitamin supplementation so widespread? The answer to this question may reside in the difficulty that parents have in determining (1) if their child would be healthier if he or she took vitamins and (2) whether their child has a nutritious diet. More realistically, the question frequently is: Does my child, who had four colds this winter, and whose diet consists primarily of mustard sandwiches and potato chips, need vitamin supplementation? These are difficult questions to answer. It is not possible to provide you with a precise way to assess the nutritional adequacy of your child's diet. We will, however, identify those exceptional situations when vitamin supplementation is necessary, and discuss the use and abuse of commonly supplemented vitamins and minerals.

## CLINICAL CONDITIONS REQUIRING VITAMIN AND MINERAL SUPPLEMENTATION

Clinically apparent vitamin deficiencies are rare in the United States. There are, however, certain clinical conditions that may require vitamin and mineral supplementation, perhaps the most common condition being premature birth. Babies born before gestation is complete have low stores of iron and are in need of iron supplementation. Depending on the degree of prematurity, supplementation with vitamins E and D, folic acid, and calcium may also be necessary.

Many physicians feel that breast-fed infants should be supplemented with vitamins C and D and iron because of borderline concentrations of these nutrients in breastmilk. Although there have been documented cases of vitamin and mineral deficiency in nursing infants, these are rare, and there are often extenuating circumstances. Many physicians (including the authors) feel that vitamin supplementation is not required in this situation.

Children who suffer from a number of illnesses causing chronic diarrhea may have difficulty absorbing vitamins that are soluble in fat, including vitamins A, D, E, and K. There are rare cases of children born with metabolic problems who require large doses of vitamins to overcome metabolic defects. An example of this is the child who develops vitamin D deficiency (rickets) with normal amounts of vitamin D, and who requires large doses to correct the problem. Some children with chronic liver diseases require vitamin A; those with chronic kidney disease may need vitamin D. Some medicines taken chronically may block the effects of particular vitamins, making vitamin supplementation necessary.

## COMMONLY SUPPLEMENTED VITAMINS

### VITAMIN A

Vitamin A is essential for growth and bone development, for vision (particularly in dim light), and for healthy skin. Human milk and infant formulas supply sufficient vitamin A for infants. Older children who eat a well-balanced diet do not need supplementation. Vitamin A in excess can cause serious health problems. Unless your physician has documented a deficiency, vitamin A should not be taken in excess of normal requirements. The effectiveness of high doses of vitamin A to improve vision, treat acne, or prevent infection is unsubstantiated and can be dangerous to your child.

## VITAMIN D

Vitamin D is important for normal bone growth and for the regulation of important minerals in the body (calcium and phosphorous). Requirements for vitamin D in healthy children are small (particularly when children are exposed to a good deal of sunlight). These requirements are almost always met by vitamin D-supplemented milk, and vitamin D-supplemented foods in the diet. Further supplementation is rarely required. Certain unusual conditions, such as inborn metabolic errors or taking antiseizure medicines, may require vitamin supplementation. The notion that vitamin D in large doses will help build stronger bones in your child is unsupported by scientific evidence; the administration of vitamin D in these large doses can have serious effects on your child.

## VITAMIN E

Vitamin E is an essential nutrient for your child. Not all its functions are well understood, but it appears to play a role in the production and integrity of red blood cells and the production of steroid hormones. It also contributes to the effectiveness of vitamin A. Nutrition surveys indicate that adequate amounts of vitamin E are supplied in a well-balanced diet. As we noted previously, premature infants have a special need for vitamin E. Children with an inability to absorb fats because of chronic diarrhea or chronic illness may require vitamin E supplementation. If your child has a balanced diet, routine vitamin E supplementation is not required. It has been claimed that high doses of vitamin E protect against heart disease, prevent cancer and mental retardation, prolong life, and increase sexual potency. There is little scientific evidence to support these claims. Large doses of vitamin E have been reported to deplete body stores of vitamins A and K. Prolonged use has also been associated with weakness, headaches, and blurred vision in some children.

## Vitamin K

Vitamin K is important for the production of factors in the blood that are responsible for clotting. Low concentrations of vitamin K in the body can lead to bleeding. Newborn infants, especially premature infants, have low levels of vitamin K and may suffer serious consequences from internal bleeding. Because of this, administration of small doses of vitamin K immediately after birth is advocated for all newborns. Some babies born at home, or in alternative birth centers, do not receive vitamin K because of parents' reluctance to have a medication and an injection interfere with the process of natural childbirth and parental attachment. Although most of these babies will do fine without vitamin K supplementation, there is a small (approximately one in two thousand newborns) chance of the occurrence of moderate to serious bleeding. Supplementation with vitamin K is not necessary after the newborn period except in children with a chronic inability to absorb fats from their instestines.

## Vitamin C

We have known for several hundred years that vitamin C is needed for normal health, and that deficiencies of vitamin C lead to serious illness—scurvy. The exact action of vitamin C in the body is not well understood. This vitamin appears to play a role in stabilizing blood vessels, in normal bone and tooth development, and in wound healing. The amount of vitamin C present in a well-balanced diet is sufficient to prevent any deficiencies. In infants who are fed cow's milk or who are on a milk-free diet, and in breast-fed infants whose mothers have insufficient intake of vitamin C, there may be a need for vitamin C supplementation. If your child's body is excessively stressed, as may occur after an operation, vitamin C supplementation may again be required. Chronic administration of certain drugs such as aspirin or phenobarbital may lead to increased losses of vitamin C and the need for supplementation. Vitamin C in large doses has been claimed to prevent and treat the common cold. Scientific studies indicate that no effect, or only a small beneficial effect, occurs with vitamin C therapy (this is discussed further in Chapter 16 on Colds). These large doses of vitamin C appear to be safe for most children. However, there have been reports of interference with vitamin $B_{12}$ and mild cases of diarrhea with these large doses.

### THE B COMPLEX VITAMINS

Deficiencies of these vitamins are rare in children who consume a normal diet. Folic acid supplementation may be required when an infant is fed primarily goat's milk. Children eating only vegetables and no dairy products or eggs may require vitamin $B_{12}$ supplementation. There is some evidence to indicate that adolescents taking oral contraceptives may need increased amounts of thiamine ($B_1$), riboflavin ($B_2$), folic acid, and vitamin $B_{12}$. Outside of these situations, there is no need for routine supplementation with B-complex vitamins.

## COMMONLY SUPPLEMENTED MINERALS

### IRON

Iron is an essential element for the production of red blood cells, and is an important component of many compounds involved with energy use in the body. Normal requirements for iron are increased in infancy, adolescence, and menstruating women. Most of your child's available iron comes from red meat and iron-fortified cereals. A small portion comes from iron-containing vegetables. Because of the lack of red meat in an infant's diet, and the low iron content of milk, children are at the greatest risk for iron deficiency during the first year of life. Iron deficiency also commonly occurs during adolescence, when there is a rapid rate of growth. Because of the danger of iron deficiency in the first year of life, many physicians recommend iron supplementation in formulas, and the use of iron-supplemented cereals for breast-fed infants. Iron status can be easily monitored with a blood test (iron deficiency will lead to a change in the size and number of red blood cells). This test is usually done at least once during childhood and adolescence. Unless your child's diet is markedly iron poor or he or she has a documented iron deficiency, we do not recommend routine iron supplementation.

### FLUORIDE

Fluoride is an important element for teeth and bone growth. It is incorporated into teeth and is felt to be important in preventing cavities. It is also felt that fluoride plays a role in building and maintaining strong bones in your child. Because supplementation with fluoride can prevent cavities, many cities have fluoridated their water supplies. If fluoridation of your water supply is less than three parts per million, supplementation with fluoride will be necessary for your child to have maximum anticavity protection. The amount of fluoride supplementation will depend on both your child's age and the amount of fluoride in the water supply. Your physician will help you in deciding whether and how much fluoride supplementation is necessary. If your child is both receiving fluoride supplementation in maximum doses and has a well-fluoridated water supply, chronic overdosage can occur, leading to a brown mottling of your child's teeth.

### TRACE ELEMENTS (COPPER, CHROMIUM, COBALT, MAGNESIUM, MOLYBDENUM, ZINC, AND SELENIUM)

It has been shown, under experimental conditions when subjects are deprived of various trace elements, that trace element deficiencies can lead to sickness. A balanced diet, however, supplies an adequate amount of trace elements for your child. During periods of stress (such as recovery from an operation or training for a marathon) supplementation may be necessary. For a child with a balanced diet we do not recommend supplementation with trace elements.

## VITAMIN AND MINERAL PREPARATIONS

Vitamin and mineral preparations are usually sold singly or in multivitamin, multimineral combinations. Combinations can be useful for specific situations such as for breast-fed infants. Here many physicians will recommend a combination of vitamins A, D, and C to supplement the borderline amount of these vitamins present in breastmilk. Other combinations may contain 50% of the recommended daily allowance of a particular vitamin (the RDA is the amount of vitamin or mineral recommended by the Food and Nutrition Board of the National Research Council to maintain good nutrition in virtually all healthy persons) and 500% of the RDA of another vitamin. You may exceed nutrient needs by several hundred percent for some vitamins and minerals in order to achieve 100% RDA for the needed nutrient. This can represent a needless expense. Preparations of liver, yeast, or wheat germ do not confer any special advantage over pure chemical preparations of vitamins and may be more expensive. Inclusion of such substances as choline, methionine, lecithin, inositol, and bioflavinoids has not been shown to be of any nutritional value. In general, we recommend that supplemental vitamins and/or minerals be given where there is a documented deficiency, or a potential risk for developing a deficiency. If it is warranted, supplementation should involve only the vitamins and minerals that are needed. Supplementation with multivitamin and multimineral preparations to correct a deficiency of one or two nutrients is excessive and expensive. Remember, excessive amounts of certain vitamins and minerals can be harmful to your child. If you have a small toddler in the house, your vitamin bottle should have a safety cap, and should be kept in a locked place. This is particularly true for candy-like preparations. Accidental poisoning with vitamin and mineral preparations can be life-threatening.

# CHAPTER THIRTEEN

# Nutrition and Behavioral Problems

MUCH HAS BEEN WRITTEN recently about the influence of nutrition on children's behavior. Three major nutritional therapies have achieved prominence in this area: (1) elimination of food additives (the Feingold diet), (2) controlling low blood sugar (hypoglycemia), and (3) the use of vitamins in large doses. Many other nutritional therapies have been advocated, but with the exception of these three therapies there is little or no scientific evidence to support or discredit these treatments. We will therefore confine our discussion and recommendations to those therapies for which some scientific information is available.

## FOOD ADDITIVES: THE FEINGOLD DIET

The Feingold diet had its origins almost ten years ago when Dr. Ben Feingold, a former director of an allergy clinic at a Kaiser Permanente Hospital in California, noted that when emotionally disturbed adults were placed on a diet free of salicylates and food additives their symptoms disappeared. He then prescribed a comparable diet for "hyperactive" children in his practice and reported that 30–50% of them became symptom free within four weeks after initiation of the diet. He published his theories in a book entitled *Why Is Your Child Hyperactive?*

In his book Feingold proposed that "hyperactive" children have a genetic "variation" that predisposes them to an abnormal reaction to food additives. He noted that salicylates and food additives do not cause allergic reactions but that they affect the body through an "innate releasing mechanism." This predisposition is felt to be permanent, and lifelong adherence to the diet is required.

For the diet to be effective, its proponents say that it must be adhered to 100%. A single bit of prohibited food can produce "hyperactivity" for three or four days, and violations of the diet occurring as infrequently as once every three or four days can completely negate the therapeutic effect of the diet. If this degree of adherence to the diet is not difficult enough, the diet itself is hard to follow. The diet dictates that most common fruits, cereals, desserts, cakes, commercial cookies, luncheon meats, soft drinks, flavored yogurts, gum, margarine, butter, candy, toothpaste, and most pediatric medications and vitamins are to be avoided. Moreover, it is recommended that the diet be followed by the whole family to avoid having prohibited foods in the house.

It is clear that adherence to the Feingold diet requires considerable energy and expense on the part of the parents. Is all this effort justified by bringing about important changes in behavior? The answer to this question depends a great deal on whom you ask. With the publication of Dr. Feingold's book, there was a proliferation of Feingold societies, groups of parents who were and still are enthusiastic supporters of the diet. The scientific community, on the other hand, reacted to the publication of the book with great skepticism. Dr. Feingold has not provided any good scientific evidence to support his theories, and many experts feel that if there are any benefits to the diet, these benefits come not from eliminating food additives but from the positive effect of cooperation among family members required for strict adherence to the diet.

In the intervening years since the introduction of the Feingold diet, several attempts have been made to prove or disprove Dr. Feingold's hypothesis. Unfortunately, the results of these studies have not done much to clear the muddied waters. In brief, some studies showed that when food additives were administered in pure form, changes in performance on a psychological test could be observed. However, when the Feingold diet was administered to a large group of children of different ages, no significant changes in performance or behavior were observed. Although the results of these scientific studies are inconclusive, there were indications in most of the studies that some individual children did respond dramatically to the salicylte- and additive-free diet. What does this all mean for you as a parent of a child with a problem with attention? It is our opinion that:

1.  there is no evidence to support the idea that food additives directly cause "hyperactivity" or any other behavior problem. If food additives do affect behavior, it is more likely that they exacerbate a pre-existing problem rather than primarily cause the problem.

2.  the Feingold diet does not take the place of more basic treatments of hyperactivity that have been previously described. It should not be used as the only form of treatment of a behavioral disorder.

3.  the Feingold diet may conceivably help your child. If you do wish to try this form of treatment, be sure that you precisely define the behaviors you wish to change so that you can more effectively evaluate the success of the diet. Also be sure to try "diet-free" intervals to see if it is diet, or some other factor, that is causing the change in behaviors.

## HYPOGLYCEMIA OR LOW BLOOD SUGAR

Hypoglycemia has been frequently invoked as a cause of behavioral problems in children. Clearly some of the manifestations of hypoglycemia are similar to characteristics seen in hyperactive children. Just as important is the fact that many important features of hypoglycemia, such as sweating, high heart rate, and fainting spells, are not seen in children with hyperactivity. Although it is conceivable that hypoglycemia can cause symptoms seen in hyperactivity, there is no scientific evidence to support any connection between low or low-normal blood sugar and changes in behavior and learning performance. The diagnosis of hypoglycemia is not easily made; it requires a five-to-seven-hour blood test called a glucose tolerance test. Even if this test turns out to be positive (a rare occurrence), it is still speculative whether the condition actually causes any behavior problems. Because of this we cannot recommend the use of a special diet to combat hypoglycemia with the hope of changing your child's behavior.

## VITAMINS AND MEGAVITAMIN THERAPY

The use of large doses of vitamins to change behavior was first practiced in the 1950s by physicians who felt that large doses of certain vitamins (nicotinic acid and nicothamide) were helpful in adults with schizophrenia. In the late 1960s, Linus Pauling, a Nobel Prize-winning biochemist, developed the concept of orthomolecular medicine. He argued that brain functioning is affected by the brain's molecular environment, and that the optimum concentration of substances such as vitamins or trace minerals present in the brain may be much higher than most people achieve with normal diet. It was hypothesized that by markedly increasing the intake of these substances the environment of the brain could be favorably changed and that this would be an effective form of treatment in mental illness. In the early 1970s this type of treatment was applied to children with learning disabilities. Unfortunately this work was not done scientifically, and it is difficult to evaluate the validity of the successful outcomes found.

Currently, the American Academy of Pediatrics does not recommend vitamin supplementation beyond the vitamins found in a well-balanced diet. The American Psychiatric Association has been more emphatic in its condemnation of orthomolecular medicine, noting that advocacy of orthomolecular treatment and megavitamins for the treatment of children with learning disabilities is unjustified. It is our opinion that there is little or no scientific evidence to recommend the use of orthomolecular treatment for treating children's behavioral problems. Although there is no harm in normal vitamin supplementation, care should be taken in giving your child megavitamin amounts (in particular vitamin A, nicotinic acid) in that they may be harmful to your child.

# CHAPTER FOURTEEN

# Immunizations

IMMUNIZATIONS HAVE undoubtedly been the most significant scientific contribution to the eradication of disease. Smallpox has been entirely eliminated from the face of the earth. Polio, which in the United States attacked 20,000 children a year in the early 1950s, now affects only a handful of children annually. Immunization campaigns, as well as legislation requiring the immunization of children before they enter school, have been responsible for the widespread implementation of immunizations. Although it is reassuring that most parents and younger physicians have never seen measles, whooping cough, or diphtheria, it is important that we do not become complacent in our immunization of children. In both Japan and England, when immunization rates for whooping cough fell in recent years, a simultaneous increase in the occurrence of whooping cough was seen.

In *Taking Care of Your Child* we discussed in detail the nature of all immunizations currently recommended for children as well as the principles of immunization therapy. In this book we shall review briefly the current recommendations for immunization of children, particularly the likelihood of reactions to the immunizations as well as some things you can do if your child develops an untoward reaction. It is beyond the scope of this book to go into a detailed discussion of the risks and benefits of each individual immunization. However, these issues have all been studied in depth, and it is our judgment, as well as the judgments of all the major policy groups concerned with immunizations, that the benefits of all the following immunizations far outweigh the associated risks. Major groups involved in these decisions include (1) the American Academy of Pediatrics, Committee on Infectious Diseases; (2) the Advisory Committee on Immunization Practices, Center for Disease Control, U.S. Public Health Service; and (3) the Council on Environmental Health, American Medical Association.

## THE DPT SHOT

The DPT shot is a single injection that provides immunity against diphtheria, pertussis (whooping cough), and tetanus. When administered according to the schedule recommended in Table 4, this series of immunizations is highly effective in preventing all these diseases. There are several hundred cases of diphtheria and tetanus reported each year. Several thousand cases of whooping cough are reported annually in the United States.

Each of the three components of the DPT immunization acts uniquely in both preventing disease and causing unwanted reactions. Diphtheria bacteria produce a toxin or poison that causes damage in humans. This toxin is altered in the

TABLE 4
IMMUNIZATIONS

| Age | Immunizations | |
|---|---|---|
| 2 MONTHS | DPT (diphtheria, pertussis, tetanus) | *and oral polio virus* |
| 4 MONTHS | DPT | |
| 6 MONTHS | DPT | *and oral polio virus* |
| 15 MONTHS | Measles, mumps, and rubella | |
| 18 MONTHS | DPT | *and oral polio virus* |
| 4–6 YEARS | DPT | *and oral polio virus* |
| EVERY 10 YEARS | Td (Tetanus and adult diphtheria) | |

laboratory to render it harmless. This harmless chemical, known as a toxoid, stimulates the body to produce a combatant chemical known as antitoxin. Although an immunized person may actually become infected with diphtheria, the dangerous toxin produced by the bacteria will be neutralized by antitoxin and the infection will do no harm. The pertussis component of the vaccine consists of killed pertussis bacteria. The formulation of this product varies from country to country and is responsible for some of the worldwide differences in reporting on the safety and efficacy of the vaccine. Most of the minor reactions that children have after a DPT injection is due to the pertussis component.

For tetanus an excellent immunization record is achieved that comes close to 100% effectiveness after the initial series of shots with a modified toxin. Local reactions are rare.

### REACTIONS TO THE DPT SHOT

Minor reactions to the DPT shot are fairly common. Over one-half of children receiving this shot will experience some form of local reaction at the site of injection, including redness, swelling, or pain. Nearly one-half of these children will have a slight fever (over 38°C or 100.4°F). About one-third will sleep more than usual; one-half will become fretful; 20% will lose their appetites for a short period of time. A much smaller percentage will either vomit or have persistent crying. Most of these reactions occur within three to six hours after the injection. If your child seems to be experiencing considerable discomfort from either the pain or high fever, we advise treating with either acetaminophen or aspirin. Most children do not require medication. We do not advise treatment for fevers less than 101.5°F.

A much smaller number of children will have more serious reactions to the DPT shot. These are usually caused by the pertussis component. A convulsion is the most common serious side effect. However, the risk of a convulsion is quite small. In a recent carefully conducted study in the United States, one in 1,750 children experienced a convulsion.

However, all these children were subsequently evaluated and found to be normal. The parents of several of these children did not even seek medical attention for the brief convulsion; this complication was detected only after a routine survey. A similar number of children lost muscle strength and became limp within 48 hours of the injection. Here again all these children were subsequently evaluated and found to be normal. The risk of permanent brain damage is unknown but estimated to be less than 1 in 100,000.

In summary, the DPT is an effective vaccine though not ideal because of the frequent minor and occasional major reactions precipitated by the pertussis component. Children who develop high temperatures (greater than 103°F) or convulsions or extreme limpness or sleepiness after one pertussis vaccination, or children who have a neurological illness or history of seizures, should not have any more. These children should instead receive the DT immunization without the P. Because pertussis is a more serious disease in infants, some physicians now question the use of pertussis booster in older children.

## POLIO

The only way to prevent polio is through immunization. There are no antibiotics that are effective against this virus. Dr. Jonas Salk introduced the inactivated polio virus vaccine (IPV) in 1955. Several years later, in 1961, the Sabin vaccine was introduced in which live polio virus was prepared in such a way as to markedly weaken it. Currently the live polio virus vaccine is administered to children orally. Because it is effective against three strains of polio virus it is also known as the triple oral polio virus vaccine (TOPV).

Side effects seen with oral polio virus vaccine are extremely rare. One or two out of 10 million vaccinated patients will develop polio. Many of those who develop polio (only about ten to twelve cases in the United States annually) are persons with rare immune diseases predisposing them to developing a wide variety of infections. Many of these patients have not even received the oral polio virus vaccine but have come in contact with individuals who were recently immunized. The injected polio virus vaccine does not seem to cause paralytic polio in these immunologically incompetent individuals. Oral polio virus vaccine is still recommended for all children except those with compromised immune systems. Breast-feeding does not interfere with the oral polio vaccine. Oral polio vaccine has not been associated with reactions such as fever or irritability.

## MMR: MEASLES, MUMPS, AND RUBELLA

It is now common practice to give the measles, mumps, and rubella vaccinations together in one shot. We shall discuss these immunizations separately. All are available as individual immunizations or in various combinations such as measles-rubella.

### MEASLES

The initial measles vaccine available in 1963 consisted of a dead virus. Many children who were immunized between 1963 and 1967 do not have adequate protection against measles, and indeed many have developed modified measles. The adolescent who was immunized before 1967 should have another measles immunization. In 1966 a weakened live virus vaccine was introduced. Although there were some initial problems, the current vaccine is far better and causes mild rash in only an estimated 5% of children and fever in approximately 10–15% of children. Here again we recommend treating fever only if it causes discomfort (generally over 101.5°F).

In years past many children were immunized at less than twelve months of age. At one year of age 10% of children receiving vaccine will not have a response and will be inadequately protected. Therefore, current recommendations are to immunize children at the age of fifteen months, when approximately 95% will receive protection. If your child was immunized at less than twelve months of age, it is advisable that he or she be reimmunized. Measles is far and away the most serious of the common childhood illnesses still encountered. We strongly urge you to check whether your child has been adequately immunized.

## MUMPS

The mumps vaccine is a live weakened virus that gives several types of protection. The most serious consequence of mumps is the inflammation of the testes and ovaries that occurs in adolescents and adults. Although these inflammations seldom produce infertility, there is considerable concern about this possibility. Mumps also produce considerable pain and discomfort when it attacks the salivary glands in the neck, producing the characteristic chipmunk-cheek appearance. The American Academy of Pediatrics recommends immunization against mumps.

## RUBELLA

Rubella immunization of children is a unique approach to preventing illness. Rubella is such a mild illness that it is virtually of no consequence to children. However, the danger lies in the risk of a pregnant woman's acquiring rubella and producing a child with severe birth defects. In 1964, during the last rubella epidemic in this country, more than 20,000 children were born with deformities caused by the rubella virus, including heart defects, blindness, and deafness.

The goal in rubella immunization is to prevent pregnant women from acquiring the disease. In 1969, the United States made a decision to attempt this by immunizing infants. Other nations adopted an alternative approach, checking preadolescent females for susceptibility to rubella and immunizing only those who had not actually developed immunity through contact with the live rubella virus. Both strategies seem to have been effective, for no major outbreaks of rubella have occurred in countries adopting either approach. However, there have been some problems with the policy of late immunization. Side effects from the rubella immunization, which are extremely rare in infants, are much more common at a later age. Particularly troublesome are the joint pains that occur in over 10% of women receiving the vaccination during adolescence or later. Some of these women had arthritis for as long as two years following immunization. In addition, a few women (between 1 in 500 and 1 in 10,000) experience a peripheral neuropathy (sensation of tingling created by inflammation in the nerves of the hands). Another risk in administering the vaccine to older women is the possibility of pregnancy at the time of vaccination. Although no birth defects have as yet occurred in pregnant women inadvertently given the rubella vaccine, vaccination is not recommended for pregnant women.

Because the reactions associated with rubella are so slight in infancy, and because rubella is combined in a single injection with the vital measles immunization, many of the debates over when to give the vaccine are more theoretical than consequential. In summary, the issues are as follows:

1. Infant boys are receiving (and their parents are being charged for) an immunization that will not benefit them but that will benefit nonimmune pregnant women who will then not be subjected to becoming infected from rubella carried by these children.

2. Because it is not entirely clear how long a rubella immunization can offer protection, it might be preferable to immunize children at an older age if they have not acquired infection naturally. However, if we had a system to routinely screen every pre-pubertal girl for the presence of antibodies capable of protecting her from rubella during pregnancy, this would be a costly procedure. In addition, those young girls who had not had rubella in the past would now be at greater risk for the side effects of the immunization.

We support the current recommendations of the American Academy of Pediatrics to immunize all children against measles, mumps, and rubella at fifteen months of age. Most schools require this immunization for admission to the first grade. Although there are theoretical reasons for supporting other immunization strategies, the testimony to our current approach is that there has not been a major rubella outbreak since 1964.

## OTHER IMMUNIZATIONS

A number of other immunizations are available, recommended for certain groups of children. Influenza virus vaccines are recommended only for children who have chronic illnesses, particularly respiratory and cardiac diseases. The pneumococcal vaccine is effective in preventing infections with this type of bacteria in children who are particularly susceptible, such as children with sickle cell disease or other disorders involving the spleen. This vaccine is effective only in children over two years of age. Hepatitis B vaccine is soon to be released and will be recommended for newborn infants born to mothers with chronic hepatitis. Vaccines are also available for rabies virus and several unusual types of bacterial infection such as meningococcal infection.

# Part III

# TREATING COMMON PROBLEMS

# CHAPTER FIFTEEN

# Fever

## DESCRIPTION

FEVER IS one of the most common symptoms of childhood, and one of the most frequent sources of anxiety for parents and of discomfort for children.

Normal body temperature differs from child to child and can vary as much as 1.5° Fahrenheit (.85° centigrade) in a healthy child during the course of a day's activities. Your child's temperature is usually at its lowest in the morning and rises during the day, especially after exercise and meals.

The most common reason for your child to have a fever is an infection. Most often that infection will involve the upper respiratory tract and will be caused by a virus. The other common causes of fever in children are sore throats, earaches, diarrhea, urinary infections, and other childhood diseases such as roseola.

Most of us know that fever is usually a sign of illness. However, one of the most common questions asked by both parents and physicians is, "Is a very high fever a sign of a very serious infection?" A high fever is not necessarily a danger sign. The vast majority of children with high fevers have a passing viral infection and will probably get better without any medical treatment within a few days. However, high fevers in certain age groups are more likely to have a serious underlying infection than those in children with a similar temperature elevation at a different age. Always consult a doctor immediately for the following circumstances:

1. fever greater than 101°F (38.3°C) in a child less than three months
2. fever greater than 103°F (39.5°C) in a child between the ages of seven and twenty-four months
3. fever greater than 105°F (41.0°C) in a child of any age
4. fever persisting for more than five days

One of the dangers of an extremely high or rapidly rising temperature is the possibility that the fever will cause a fever fit or seizure called a *febrile convulsion*. These seizures are relatively common in normal healthy children; about 3–5% will experience one. Unfortunately, it is impossible to predict or prevent febrile seizures. Even though most are of no consequence, these seizures are one of the most frightening things for a parent to experience. This topic is discussed further in *Taking Care of Your Child*.

### RATIONALE FOR TREATMENT

Although there are a few scientists who argue that fever may be beneficial—and indeed some rare diseases are even treated with fever therapy—we recommend treatment of fevers over 101°F (38.3°C) because this degree of fever makes most children feel uncomfortable. Because most febrile seizures occur during the first part of an illness when the fever is rising, they are difficult to prevent with aspirin or acetaminophen. Bringing your child's fever down will make him or her comfortable, but it will not change the course of the illness, and it may or may not prevent febrile seizures.

### HOME TREATMENT

There is nothing your doctor can do for reducing a fever that you cannot do at home. A doctor's visit is often necessary to determine the underlying infection responsible for the fever, but you can treat your child's fever just as easily as your doctor can.

The first decision is whether to treat it or not. Remember, many children run temperatures up to 100.4°F normally. Rectal temperatures are more reliable and generally run

0.5°F higher than oral temperatures. Underarm temperatures are somewhat cumbersome to take; plastic strips placed
on a child's forehead are inaccurate. Discomfort is the main
reason for attempting to lower a fever. Many children will
begin to feel uncomfortable over a temperature of 101°F;
most children will be noticeably affected over 102°F.
Once you have decided to treat the temperature yourself,
you have several choices. Even though countless remedies
have been suggested, only a few have been proved effective.
Some methods, however, can be far more dangerous than the
fever. For example, never try to bring your child's temperature down by rubbing with alcohol, for the alcohol fumes can
irritate your child's lungs. Similarly, ice baths cause considerable discomfort. Never bathe your child in ice water; the
purpose of the therapy is to make the child more comfortable! Sponging or bathing your child in lukewarm water is
effective in bringing very high fevers down to approximately
102°F (39°C). However, sometimes the inside of the body
responds to this external cooling by a compensating mechanism that may tend to elevate the temperature. Another approach shown to be effective, though not widely utilized, is
massage. Massage stimulates the skin and causes an expan-
sion of the blood vessels near the skin surface that allows
heat to dissipate through the skin.
The mainstay of fever reduction is treatment with either
aspirin or acetaminophen. Both agents have been shown to
be equally effective when given in appropriate therapeutic
dosages. The safety of these products, however, differs. The
principal problems with aspirin include the irritating action
on the stomach's lining as well as the potential for interfering
with the clotting properties of the blood. In overdoses aspirin
causes a buildup of body acids in the blood that may cause
severe illness and even death. Although safety caps have
markedly reduced the number of fatal accidental ingestions
from aspirin, massive overdoses and deaths still occur. However, given its widespread and longstanding use, in therapeutic doses aspirin is a remarkably safe drug. There have been
several recent reports in which aspirin has been associated

with a serious and often fatal condition known as Reye's syndrome. This syndrome is extremely rare—only 200–500 cases occur annually in the United States. The syndrome has also been associated with influenza and chicken pox infections. Because the relationship between aspirin and this rare syndrome is still unclear, several notes of caution have recently been published. Parents are advised that, when possible, aspirin should be avoided for children with chicken pox and during influenza-like illnesses.

Acetaminophen has remarkably few adverse or side effects at therapeutic dosages. However, massive overdoses can result in severe liver damage and even death. Although numerous deaths have resulted from suicidal ingestions of acetaminophen, at the time of this writing only one childhood death has been reported in the United States.

In short, both aspirin and acetaminophen are quite safe in therapeutic dosages and they are of equivalent efficacy. Acetaminophen seems to have a somewhat greater safety margin and for this reason we generally recommend it slightly over aspirin as the first drug with which to start. An additional advantage to acetaminophen, beyond its slight margin of safety, is the fact that it comes in liquid preparations whereas aspirin does not come in liquid form. A word of caution, however. Acetaminophen also comes in drops that contain more than three times as much acetaminophen as the elixir. It is important not to confuse these different preparations. If your doctor advises that you give your two-year-old a teaspoon of acetaminophen, he or she is really talking about the elixir; he or she would most likely tell you to give your two-year-old two dropperfulls of the acetaminophen drops.

If either acetaminophen or aspirin does not lower your child's temperature, you can combine the two. Studies have shown that combining these two different drugs causes both a greater and a more prolonged drop in children's fevers. There is an added advantage. When combined, the drugs need be given together only every six hours. Although many physicians recommend alternating acetaminophen with aspirin on an every-two-hour basis, this regimen has never been clinically compared to these other regimens, is inconvenient, and can be confusing to boot. We do not recommend it.

## TREATMENT AFTER CONSULTING YOUR PHYSICIAN

Aspirin and acetaminophen are the only medications used to reduce fever in children. Both are available without prescription. Although other medications can reduce fever, their use is generally directed toward children with problems such as rheumatoid arthritis, and these medications are not specifically intended for fever reduction.

## IS THE TREATMENT WORKING?

The duration of fever really depends on the nature of the underlying infection. Most minor colds accompanied by fever pass in two to three days; fever present for longer than five days should prompt a contact with your physician. A fever that is easily reduced by acetaminophen or aspirin does not necessarily signify that there is no serious underlying problem. Always look at your child and not at your child's thermometer. If, despite therapeutic doses of acetaminophen and aspirin combined, your child continues to have a fever that is causing discomfort, you should contact your physician.

Many children are incapable of taking aspirin. If your child has acute stomach cramps following aspirin, you should consider using buffered aspirin. If this still does not alleviate the symptoms, you should consider eliminating aspirin from your therapeutic repertoire. Some children may also develop wheezing following aspirin. Again, if this happens to your child you should refrain from using aspirin.

# CHAPTER SIXTEEN

# The Cold: *Nasal Congestion, Cough, Earache*

COLDS TO MOST PARENTS mean fevers, runny noses, coughs, and irritable and grumpy children. To some parents, colds may also mean vomiting, diarrhea, and even rashes. This wide variation in the understanding of what a cold is can lead to problems in using medicines in the home treatment of colds. When your physician prescribes medicines for colds, he or she usually has a specific illness in mind, and a specific set of symptoms. Unless you understand this definition, it will be difficult for you to evaluate the effectiveness and the utility of the prescribed treatments.

For most physicians, a *cold* is an infection caused by a virus that involves the nose, throat, and sometimes the large airways of the lungs. A cold does not involve the stomach, the gut, the skin, or other parts of the body, nor is it an allergy. A cold should also not be confused with the conditions that may result from a cold. These can include ear infections (otitis media), sinus infection (sinusitis), and lung infections (pneumonia). This distinction is important because these conditions demand different treatments and medicines. Some physicians also reserve the term *flu* for more serious infections of the nose, throat, and lungs and their airways caused by a specific virus, the influenza virus. This infection occurs in epidemics in the winter months; it can cause serious problems for children who are at risk, and it can be prevented by a vaccine. Although some physicians use the term flu loosely for all colds, for our purposes we will not include this specific infection in our discussion.

Let us return to our definition of a cold. First, we said that a cold is an *infection* caused by a *virus*. Because the cold is an infection, and a minor infection at that, it is a self-limited illness. This means that in a short period of time your child's body will be able to mount an attack against the virus and eliminate the infection. How short or long this time is depends to a large extent on your child's age. For an infant, it is not unusual for a cold to last several weeks; an adolescent, however, may be over his or her cold in four to five days.

Because colds are caused by viruses, they cannot be treated with antibiotics. In fact, there are no safe, easily available medicines that can kill a virus. This means that no matter what treatment or medicine you give, a cold will get better in a short period of time. Any medicine or treatment you do give may help alleviate the symptoms of a cold, but it will not shorten the period of time it takes your body to fight off that cold.

Colds in children are frequently accompanied by fever, fatigue, achiness, fatiguability, and grumpiness. This may manifest itself in your child being unwilling to follow instructions, do schoolwork, sustain any interest while playing, and in general demanding that you be at their side constantly.

Your physician has little to offer for relief of these symptoms beyond your tender loving care. If your child's cold should cause marked swings in behavior, with either extreme irritability and grumpiness or extreme lethargy and listlessness, your physician should be contacted, for this may indicate the onset of a more serious illness.

When your child has a bad cold, there is no question that he or she will want extra attention. Your best bet in this situation is to give your child as much attention and affection as is possible. This will allow your child to feel that his or her needs are being met during a stressful period, leading to a secure feeling and an enhanced sense of well-being. Do not worry about spoiling your child. Return to previously established limits of behavior can be quickly accomplished after the cold is over. Giving your child acetaminophen or aspirin in this situation may be helpful. You do not have to wait until a fever is present to give your child these medicines.

Fortunately for parents almost all treatment of colds can be accomplished at home with medicines available over the counter without a physician's prescription. It is useful in discussing the home treatment of colds to consider the symptoms one by one. For fever see Chapter 15.

## NASAL CONGESTION

### DESCRIPTION

These symptoms are caused by a direct effort of the cold virus on the nose and its blood vessels. When the virus attacks the nose it causes certain cells in the nose to give off increased amounts of mucus, and it causes the blood vessels of that nose to become congested or to fill up with blood. This causes mucus to drip from the nose and for the nose to swell shut from the congested blood vessels. Some of these effects are mediated by chemicals that travel from cell to cell and from cell to blood vessel. One important class of these chemicals is the histamines.

### RATIONALE FOR TREATMENT

Treatment to alleviate the symptoms of a runny nose and nasal congestion is aimed at (1) shrinking the blood vessels or *decongesting* them, and (2) blocking the chemicals that mediate the symptoms in the nose. The medicines that may accomplish this fall into two major categories: decongestants and antihistamines.

*Decongestants* Decongestants shrink the size of the blood vessels in the nose, decrease the swelling, and make it easier to breathe. There are three major classes of decongestants. The first class, which includes pseudoephedrine and ephedrine, can be given as a nasal spray, as a pill, or as liquid. The effects of these medicines generally last six to eight hours with the major effects occurring in the first one to two hours. When these medicines are given by mouth, they affect the rest of the body as well as the nose. This is most evident to you in changes in your child's behavior. These medicines can cause an increase in the general activity level of your child, or as some parents say, "It makes him hyper" or "She gets wired on this medicine." Paradoxically, these medicines can also make your child sleepy or listless. It is difficult to predict how your child will react. It is prudent, however, to try these medicines during the "easy" part of the day to determine what the effect will be. It is unfortunate to discover at ten o'clock at night that your child's activity level has markedly increased with these medicines.

When these medicines are given by nasal spray, the effects on the rest of the body are much less marked. There are, however, problems with this route of administration. Although the actions of the medication are rapid and effective in the spray form, when the effect wears off the nasal congestion often returns more severely than before, a phenomenon called *rebound*. After a while the nose spray needs to be used with increasing frequency to alleviate the symptoms. This can cause an inflammation of the nose (rhinitis medicamentosa) and more congestion. This vicious cycle can lead to an addiction to the nasal spray. To avoid this, you must be careful to limit use to two to three days, and you must be sure to follow the recommended dosing schedule.

Phenylpropanolamine is another class of decongestant found in many cold preparations (such as Dimetapp) that can be given by mouth; its effect can last up to six hours. Phenylpropanolamine has the same side effects on your child as those described for ephedrine and pseudoephedrine. This medicine has also been used in adults as an appetite suppressant and may exert a similar effect in children. It also has been found to cause elevated blood pressure in some adults at prescribed doses. This effect has not, however, been documented in children.

The third class of commonly prescribed decongestants consists of oxymetazoline and xylometazoline (for example, Afrin). These medicines are administered only in a nasal spray. They have the advantage of a long duration of action of up to eight to twelve hours. These decongestants have minimal effects on the rest of the body; but they cause serious rebound congestion when withdrawn. Caution should be exercised not to use these medicines for more than three days and at no greater dosing frequency than once every twelve hours.

The effectiveness of decongestants is a hotly debated topic. There is no question that the administration of these medicines by nasal spray or drops makes it easier to breathe through the nose. Their effectiveness in drying up a runny nose is less impressive. Again, these potentially beneficial effects must be balanced against the problem of rebound. When these medicines are given by mouth, there is even greater controversy as to whether they make it easier to breathe or dry up a runny nose. Some scientific studies have shown that these decongestants work, whereas other studies have shown no effect at all from their use. It is difficult to make sweeping conclusions about the effectiveness of oral decongestants for all children. What every parent should do is watch the child closely and see if the medicine markedly increases the ease of breathing or decreases the running nose. Without a marked effect, we feel that oral decongestants are not worth the side effects that usually accompany their use.

*Antihistamines*  Antihistamines are the second major group of medicines used to treat nasal congestion and runny noses. Although there are a myriad of antihistamine preparations on the market, all have been designed to block the effect of histamines on congestion of blood vessels and the production of mucus secretions in the nose. Antihistamines have been shown effective in decongesting the blood vessels of the nose in allergic conditions; their effectiveness in decreasing nasal congestion in a cold is less certain. Antihistamines appear to decrease nasal secretions in a cold and aid in drying up the runny nose. Antihistamines have also been used to prevent ear infections and the accumulation of fluid behind the eardrum during a cold. There is now good evidence, however, that they are not effective for this purpose.

To summarize, antihistamines may be effective in drying up nasal secretions in a cold, and are only questionably effective in increasing nasal breathing during the cold. They do not appear to be effective in preventing ear infections or the accumulation of fluid behind the eardrum.

Antihistamines have many side effects. Fortunately, the serious side effects are rare. The less serious side effects are common and need to be anticipated. For most children, the administration of antihistamines will bring about drowsiness and listlessness. When given to an irritable, crying child at bedtime this drowsiness can help relax the child, increase the amount of sleep he or she gets, and in certain situations preserve his or her parents' sanity. On the other hand, when these medicines are given before school the resulting drowsiness may seriously compromise the child's effort that day. The degree of drowsiness varies among the types of antihistamines used. If drowsiness is a problem, this should be discussed with your physician, who may want to select another type of antihistamine. Some children may react paradoxically to antihistamines, and instead of becoming drowsy these children may experience nervousness, increased activity, and difficulty in falling asleep. Unfortunately there is no way to predict in advance what will happen; you have to try out the antihistamines to determine the individual effects on your child. Children taking an antihistamine can also commonly experience a dry nose, mouth, and throat, and loss of appetite. The degree of these effects again varies from child to child.

When purchasing antihistamine preparations in the drug store you are confronted with a tremendous number of different cold preparations containing different classes of antihistamines as well as antihistamines in combination with decongestants. The description of these common classes of antihistamines, some representatives of those classes, and their most commonly encountered side effects can be found in Part D of this book. It has not been documented that one class or type of antihistamine is more effective than another in alleviating the nasal symptoms of the cold. The choice of antihistamine will depend more on the type of preparation desired, that is, with or without the decongestant effect or with long- or short-term action, and on the side effects experienced by the individual child. As was previously mentioned, antihistamines are frequently combined with decongestants in the same cold medicine. This combination has the theoretical advantages (1) that it will significantly affect both increased nasal congestion and increased nasal secretions, and (2) that the decongestant will counteract the drowsiness caused by the antihistamine. However, there are no studies available to prove or disprove these suppositions. Moreover, the use of two drugs increases the chance of significant side effects. Again, decisions as to what type of cold medicine to use to alleviate nasal symptoms are best made after observing the effects of a particular preparation on your child and discussing this with his or her physician. Some medicines will also combine more than one type of antihistamine. The hope here is that the combination will increase the effectiveness of the preparation without increasing the side effects, but no evidence proves or disproves this outcome in children with colds.

## OTHER HOME TREATMENT

Use of a vaporizer or placing your child in a hot steamy bathroom serves to moisten the airway and to loosen up the mucus inside, making it easier to blow out. This is particularly useful when the humidity is low in your house and the mucus in the nose becomes dry and impacted. A vaporizer serves to keep the air moist and the secretions loose on a constant basis. It is best to use a cool mist vaporizer, for a hot-water humidifier has the potential of burning young children should they improperly handle the heater. A hot, steamy bathroom can also loosen mucus in the nose, but it has the disadvantage of being intermittent rather than constant in its effect.

Mentholated rubs have been used for years by parents to ease breathing and nasal congestion. They are usually applied to the chest or under the nose, or put on the pillow. There is scant scientific evidence to show that they are effective in alleviating nasal congestion. However, this is not to say that they do not make children feel better. Although their effects have been poorly studied and it is difficult to conclude exactly what they accomplish, it is equally difficult to deny the beneficial effect of the sense of well-being that accompanies a mother gently rubbing the salve on a child's chest. This alone may make the treatment worthwhile.

Believe it or not, chicken soup has been subjected to scientific scrutiny and is effective in altering the flow of mucus in a way which may be helpful. The heat of the chicken soup may be the key factor, but we recommend this traditional culinary remedy because of its good taste and safety.

## IS THE TREATMENT WORKING?

If these medicines are making nasal breathing easier, you should notice less need for mouth-breathing. This is best assessed at night or during naptime, when you can see if your child is breathing with his or her mouth open. For the younger infant, increased nasal breathing will mean an easier time with nursing or taking a bottle. When the infant can breathe through the nose, he or she does not need to stop feeding to gulp air and will not be as frustrated with feeding. You may also be able to notice more subtle changes such as less drooling in the infant or decreased nasal speech in the older child. Most parents can detect a decrease in the runniness of the nose by noticing how frequently they wipe their child's nose and the amount of sniffling that takes place. The amount of "noisy breathing" that occurs when the child is sleeping may also be an indicator of how the medicine is working. As will be discussed later, you may also notice a decrease in the amount of nighttime coughing. Again, it is important that you perceive significant improvements in your child's symptoms before you subject him or her to the common and unpleasant side effects of these medicines.

## COUGH
### DESCRIPTION

The cough that comes with a cold is caused by two different mechanisms. First, cold viruses can directly infect the back of the throat, the voice box, and the large airways of the lungs. This will lead to inflammation, irritation, and the production of mucus in these locations. The cough is a response by the body designed to prevent the mucus secretions from getting into the lungs and possibly causing pneumonia. Occasionally a cough from a cold will persist even after excess mucus production has subsided; this comes from residual inflammation causing a "tickle in the throat" that may last for up to two to three weeks following the disappearance of other symptoms. The more common mechanism of producing a cough during a cold is the dripping of nasal secretions back down the throat when your child is lying down. When this occurs, your child coughs up the secretions before they settle in the lungs, a condition commonly called *postnasal drip*. In both cases, the cough represents a protective response of the body that must be taken into consideration when determining how zealous to be in suppressing the cough.

### RATIONALE FOR TREATMENT

In general, when a cough is sufficiently frequent and troublesome that it keeps you and your child awake for most of the night, this is an indication for the use of cough suppressants. Here the importance of a good night's sleep for both you and your child outweighs any potential disadvantages in suppressing the cough. Occasionally a cough may be sufficiently severe that it interferes with the daily activities of eating, playing, and school work. Here again a cough suppressant is indicated to return life to normal for you and your child.

### HOME TREATMENT

Like nasal congestion and a runny nose, a cough caused by a cold can be treated at home with the use of medicines that are available over the counter without a doctor's prescription. If the cough is due to direct irritation of the throat and the airways, there are several medicines available in your pharmacy for suppression of cough. The most commonly used medicine and one of the most effective is dextromethorphan hydrobromide. This is a nonnarcotic medicine that suppresses a cough by acting on cough centers in the brain. Because of its nonnarcotic nature, it can be used around the clock without the fear of behavioral changes or addiction. Scientific studies have shown that the cough suppressant effect of dextromethorphan hydrobromide is equivalent to that of more powerful narcotic cough suppressors such as codeine. Codeine, however, does have a sedative and calming effect on your child that may play a part in suppressing a cough and increasing your child's sense of well-being. Antihistamines are another class of medicines that have been advertised as being effective in a cough caused by a cold. They are thought to be effective because of their ability to partially numb the back of the throat and relieve the tickle that provokes the cough. There is also some evidence that some antihistamines, in particular diphenhydramine hydrochloride (Benadryl, Benylin), may also act directly on the cough center in the brain to suppress the cough.

The third medicine that is commonly available over the counter to suppress coughs is guaifenesin (such as Robitussin). This medicine is supposed to loosen up the secretions in the large airways of the lung and make them easier to cough up. Once the secretions have been effectively eliminated, the need to cough will hopefully disappear. There is good evidence, however, that this medicine is no more effective than honey lemon tea for this purpose and probably not as soothing. A variety of cough drops are also sold over the counter to suppress the cough of a cold. They work by partially numbing the back of the throat and reducing the amount of tickle. Some cough drops do contain dextromethorphan hydrobromide as well as the soothing and numbing agents. For some children, cough drops do make the back of the throat feel cool and more comfortable. This alone can increase your child's sense of well-being and reduce the anxiety that often provokes repeated coughing attacks.

If the cough is due to a postnasal drip, an antihistamine is the indicated medicine because of its ability to dry up the secretions in the nose and prevent them from dripping back down the throat. Again, because of the common behavioral changes associated with it, this medicine is best confined to use at bedtime, when a cough secondary to postnasal drip is most troublesome. A cough associated with a cold may frequently be caused by both direct irritation and postnasal drip, or it may be difficult for you to decide what is happening. Here it may be advisable to buy a cough medicine that acts against both types of cough.

## TREATMENT AFTER CONSULTING YOUR PHYSICIAN

The major medicine available to your physician for suppressing coughs is codeine, which suppresses all types of cough by acting on the centers in the brain that trigger the cough response. Codeine can be particularly useful for the dry cough that persists after a cold, or for coughing spells that occur from a tickly throat. It is, however, a narcotic with a sedative effect and with a potential for addiction. Because of this, it is advisable to limit its use to nighttime, when the behavioral changes will be less troublesome and when the cough is most disabling. Again, there is little evidence to suggest that codeine is any more effective a cough suppressant than is dextromethorphan hydrobromide. However, it does have the advantage of a sedative and calming effect that can significantly contribute to reducing the anxiety that is associated with coughing and that in itself may provoke more coughing. We suggest, however, that you try nonnarcotic cough suppressants such as dextromethorphan hydrobromide or antihistamines before turning to a codeine preparation for help.

It is important to realize that a cough can on occasion be a symptom of more than just a cold. If your child's cough worsens during a cold and if the cough produces a yellow sputum and is associated with an increase in fever, your child may be developing pneumonia. In this situation it is important that you call your physician to determine if your child needs to be examined for this possibility. If your child does have pneumonia, antibiotics may be employed to eliminate the bacteria in the lungs that are causing the irritation and producing the cough.

In summary, the cough associated with a cold is a protective mechanism to prevent the cold from settling into the lungs. In some instances, the cough can become a significant symptom that keeps your child awake, disturbs his or her schoolwork, makes it difficult for him or her to eat, or just drives him or her to distraction. When this occurs, it may be advisable to treat the cough. There is no advantage in treating a cough that does not significantly bother your child; in fact there may be harm done by the side effects of the medicine. Your physician can be of assistance to you in helping you to make this decision.

### Is the Treatment Working?

Most cough suppressant medicines have a fairly rapid onset of action, and you should notice an effect within one or two hours. If you do not see a reduction in the amount of coughing, this may be because that particular cough preparation chosen does not work for your child, or it may indicate that the cough is due to more than a cold—for example, to pneumonia. However, this latter possibility is rare; in addition, it is usually associated with fever and a cough that produces yellow sputum. If you do not see any improvement, stop the medicine. Some children, for reasons we do not know, will not respond to cough suppressants. If this is the case you can grin and bear it until the cold resolves, or you can consult your physician about another cough medicine.

## EARACHES
### Description

Earache associated with a cold is a common problem that is usually due to the accumulation of fluid behind the eardrum in the middle ear. This is sometimes referred to as *serous otitis media*. Occasionally this accumulation of fluid can lead to a middle-ear infection that is called *otitis media*. When this occurs, your child will usually complain of intense ear pain and you will notice fever, listlessness, or irritability. If this occurs during a cold, you should contact your physician for possible treatment (see Chapter 18, Ear Problems).

### RATIONALE FOR TREATMENT

The presence of fluid in the middle ear may cause a dull earache in your child and a decrease or dullness to his or her hearing. It was felt at one time that the use of decongestants and/or antihistamines could prevent the accumulation of fluid in the middle ear. Recent research, however, has shown that antihistamines and decongestants do not prevent the development of serous otitis media, and that these medicines should not be used for this purpose.

### HOME TREATMENT

There is little that can be done at home to prevent or to treat the accumulation of fluid in the middle ear. Acetaminophen or aspirin can be given to alleviate pain. If the symptoms persist for more than two weeks after the cold has disappeared, your physician should be consulted.

### TREATMENT AFTER CONSULTING YOUR PHYSICIAN

There is little your physician can do to prevent or treat serous otitis media. However, if the symptoms persist for more than two weeks, he or she may want to examine your child's ears and follow the situation closely to see that the fluid does disappear. Persistence of the fluid over a long period of time may affect your child's hearing and in the young child may affect language development. If the fluid persists for more than six weeks, your physician may want to consider making an opening in the ear drum to release fluid and/or inserting tubes between the middle ear and the outer ear to make sure that fluid does not reaccumulate.

## SORE THROAT

### DESCRIPTION

Sore throat associated with a cold may be due to irritation and inflammation caused by the cold virus, or it may be due to dryness and irritation from the mouth-breathing that accompanies nasal congestion. See Chapter 17, Sore Throats.

### HOME TREATMENT

If the sore throat is caused by irritation from the cold virus, acetaminophen or aspirin can be of use in alleviating the pain. Various gargles are available over the counter but in general these have not been helpful in children. If the sore throat is caused by persistent mouth-breathing, decongestants that open up the nasal airways and antihistamines that dry up the secretions may be helpful. Again, because sore throats associated with colds have both mechanisms involved, it may be prudent to combine these medicines for effective relief.

### IS THE TREATMENT WORKING?

If acetaminophen or aspirin is used to alleviate the pain, you should see some reduction in symptoms within one to two hours. If antihistamines or decongestants are employed to alleviate nasal congestion, some effects should be seen after a night's sleep without mouth-breathing.

### PREVENTION

A final word should be said about the prevention of colds. As we have said previously, antibiotics have no role in the treatment of colds. They are not effective in killing the viruses that cause colds and as such cannot be used to prevent colds or to treat colds. The use of antibiotics to prevent your child from getting a cold is not only ineffective, but may potentially be harmful. Much has been written about the use of vitamins in the prevention and treatment of colds, in particular, large doses of vitamin C. Like most controversial issues in medicine, both supporters and detractors of the use of vitamin C are found in abundance. A few things, however, can be said with some clarity about vitamin C. First, in the doses recommended by most proponents, vitamin C does not appear to be harmful. Second, in most of the careful studies done on the effectiveness of vitamin C in preventing and treating colds, there were either no differences between users and nonusers of vitamin C in the number and duration of colds; any differences were small. Because of the questionable beneficial effect of vitamin C, it is difficult to make a wholesale recommendation of this form of treatment. On the other hand, this therapy is not harmful and therefore it is difficult to condemn its use. In the end, we are left with giving you yet another opinion about vitamin C; it is our opinion that vitamin C is not harmful but is not significantly effective in the prevention or treatment of colds. Because of this lack of effectiveness, we do not recommend the use of vitamin C for these purposes.

# CHAPTER SEVENTEEN

# Pharyngitis: *Sore Throat*

## DESCRIPTION

CHILDREN ARE BROUGHT to physicians more often for sore throat than for any other problem or symptom. Physicians make a diagnosis of pharyngitis or tonsillitis over 12,000,000 times a year in persons less than twenty-one years old. An additional twelve to sixteen million sore throats are estimated to be managed entirely at home.

Although when a child complains of soreness in his or her throat, that child may actually have an irritation in the airways or more seriously in the opening to the airway (the epiglottis), soreness when swallowing generally means an irritation of the throat and/or the tonsils. A wide variety of noninfectious and infectious agents are responsible; viruses cause the majority of cases. Although all invading agents can cause the annoying symptoms of soreness, difficulty in swallowing, headache, and fever, only bacterial infections have consequences that are detrimental to a child's health. The vast majority of bacterial infections in children are caused by group A beta-hemolytic streptococci, which cause a condition known as *strep throat*. The consequences of strep throat, in addition to annoying symptoms, are principally of two types. Local bacterial infections can occur, including pus in the throat and around the tonsils as well as mastoiditis (infection of the bone behind the ear). These complications are extremely rare. In addition, a strep throat can lead to a kidney problem known as glomerulonephritis ten to fourteen days after the infection begins, or rheumatic fever three to four weeks after the infection begins. Although rheumatic fever was a significant problem in the past, afflicting as many as 3% of patients with strep throat, it is much less of a problem today, attacking only about one in one thousand patients with strep throat. Some individuals, however, may be more susceptible to rheumatic fever than are the majority.

Because neither you nor your physician can tell a viral sore throat from a strep throat, and because the complications of strep throat continue to affect some children, we advise a visit to your physician for a throat culture in all children in whom the symptom persists for more than several hours.

### RATIONALE FOR TREATMENT

A major basis for the antibiotic treatment of a sore throat is to prevent a streptococcal infection from causing rheumatic fever. This treatment will also probably prevent the occurrence of rare infectious complications such as mastoiditis. Studies have shown that penicillin most probably does not have any effect on altering the course of your child's symptoms. Because delaying treatment for twenty-four to forty-eight hours will not reduce the ability of penicillin to prevent rheumatic fever, there is no additional risk to your child while waiting the results of a throat culture. Because over 80% of sore throats are due to viruses, awaiting throat culture results will most often protect your child from experiencing any side effects of antibiotics, which, after all, are unnecessary for the overwhelming majority of sore throats. Many parents are concerned about withholding antibiotics while waiting the throat culture results. However, because penicillin does not relieve symptoms, it is important to turn your attention to other remedies that might be effective in reducing symptoms. Remember, withholding antibiotics is not the same as withholding treatment.

### HOME TREATMENT

Many items are available to help relieve your child's sore throat symptoms. If fever is present, we recommend either acetaminophen or aspirin, both of which are also effective in reducing pain. Most children will find cold liquids that are neither acidic nor bubbly to be soothing. This is a good time for cold juices, or even popsicles or ice cream. Over the years we have heard of countless home remedies, many of which pose risks seemingly as great as the infection itself. Most parents do not need to be told to avoid kerosene-soaked rags around their child's throat. It is best to avoid most elaborate concoctions. Salt-water gargles are simple and safe enough. Add one-half teaspoon salt to an eight-ounce glass of water. Be sure that your child does not complain that this treatment is worse than the illness. Mouthwashes and gargles do not have an antibacterial effect, but they may soothe soreness. However, no studies have been conducted demonstrating their effectiveness. Several over-the-counter preparations are available that include the mild anesthetic phenol (Cepastat, Chloraseptic) or cooling agents such as menthol (Vicks Throat Lozenges.) Phenol can be irritating in doses high enough to relieve pain; menthol appears safe but has not been demonstrated to be superior to other cooling liquids available in the refrigerator. We feel that these preparations do not offer any advantage over salt-water gargles or cool liquids, and we do not recommend them routinely.

### TREATMENT AFTER CONSULTING YOUR PHYSICIAN

If your child is diagnosed as having strep throat, a full ten-day course of antibiotics will be given. Penicillin is the drug of choice except for children who are allergic to penicillin; erythromycin is then substituted. One penicillin injection with benzathine penicillin is effective. This is a long-acting form of penicillin and only one shot is necessary. The alternative treatment is taking either phenoxymethyl penicillin or penicillin G four times daily for ten days. Failure to take the medication for this duration of time may not fully eradicate the infection. For older children this is a situation where you may offer a choice. An injection is certainly painful, but it is over quickly and it avoids the problems that go along with having to remember to take forty doses of medication. Over the years it has been surprising how many children have opted for taking one shot to "get it over with."

### Is the Treatment Working?

The symptoms of a strep throat, including fever, generally last for about five days whether or not the antibiotic therapy is being given. If the fever persists for longer than five days your physician should be contacted as the infection may be spreading. Persistent difficulty in swallowing should also prompt a call to your physician. Drooling is a sign either that an abscess may be forming or that the child's breathing passages may be involved. Drooling or a decrease in your child's ability to speak should prompt you to seek immediate medical attention.

The kidney disturbance that may follow a strep throat cannot be prevented by antibiotics. You will recognize its occurrence because your child's urine will become a dark cola color. He or she may also experience swelling of the eyelids or severe headaches. Rheumatic fever generally begins with joint pain and fever, and may be seen with one of several unusual skin reactions. Fortunately, both of these complications are rare.

Scarlet fever is nothing more than a strep throat with a red skin rash. It is no more serious than a regular strep throat. Because it is easy to recognize, your physician will undoubtedly begin antibiotic treatment as soon as he or she makes a diagnosis. The fever should go away within three days. The rash, however, may persist for several weeks and may even cause a sunburn-like peeling on the palms. This is not cause for alarm, for it is part of the natural progress of this illness.

# CHAPTER EIGHTEEN

# Ear Problems: *Otitis Media, Otitis Externa*

By Benjamin Goodman, Jr., M.D. *

AN EARACHE IS ONE of the most common problems seen in children. The usual causes are infections of the middle ear (otitis media) or of the outer portion of the ear canal (otitis externa). Ear pain may also result from differences in pressure between the external ear and the middle ear such as may occur during ascent and descent in an airplane, or it may be a pain referred from another part of the mouth or face, such as the teeth. In this chapter, we will confine most of our discussion to infections in the middle ear and the external ear.

## OTITIS MEDIA

### DESCRIPTION

Middle-ear infections are probably the most common infectious disease seen in children. Within the first three years of life over 71% of children will experience at least one episode of otitis media. In over 40% of these children a second episode will occur. These episodes usually follow a cold but may occur with allergy or with no known cause. Middle-ear infections result from a malfunctioning of the drainage tube (eustachian tube) from the middle ear to the back of the mouth. This leads to an accumulation in the middle ear of fluid and bacteria—the primary ingredients for an infection. Colds lead to ear infections because the swollen lymph tissue or glands in the back of the throat may block these drainage tubes and interfere with the normal clearance of fluid and

* Associate Professor, Department of Family Medicine, Medical University of South Carolina.

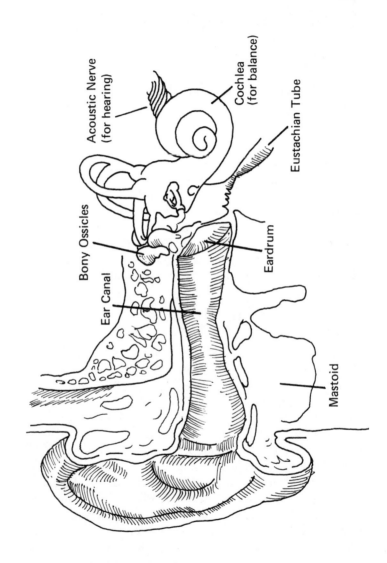

equalization of pressure between the middle ear and the mouth. Feeding an infant in the supine position (often by propping up the bottle) may force fluid up through the drainage tubes into the middle ear during swallowing and predispose to ear infections. Allergic conditions may cause swelling and blockage of the drainage tubes and can also lead to an accumulation of fluid in the middle ear. This fluid provides an excellent breeding ground for bacteria and greatly increases the chance of an ear infection in your child. Fortunately, the number of ear infections a child will get in one year decreases rapidly after the age of three years. This may be due to a better functioning of the drainage tubes or an increased ability on the part of the child to fight colds. Recovering from an ear infection can be a long process. After an ear infection, 40% of children will have persistent fluid in the middle ear for up to four weeks, and 10% of children will have fluid in the middle ear for at least three months. Presence of this fluid may cause a mild decrease in hearing and some ear discomfort.

### RATIONALE FOR TREATMENT

Physicians treat middle-ear infections to decrease pain and discomfort in the child and to avoid scarring and permanent damage to the eardrum. Treatment of the middle-ear infection also prevents the further spread of bacteria to other parts of the body and more serious infections. Unfortunately, treatment with antibiotics does not always accomplish these goals. Children who are treated after the infection has been present for several days, and some older children in general, may not respond quickly or at all to a course of antibiotics. Most physicians feel that the treatment with antibiotics decreases the possibility of scarring and permanent damage to the eardrum; however, there are children who have been adequately treated with antibiotics for their acute middle-ear infection who still have sustained damage to their eardrums. Treatment of middle-ear infections with antibiotics most probably prevents other serious infections, but there is no clear cut scientific proof of this fact. Although antibiotic treatment is not 100% effective for all children with middle-ear infections it is the best treatment we have, and for most children it will result in rapid improvement in the symptoms and resolution of the ear infection without problems. It would be nice to be able to prevent the accumulation of fluid in the middle ear after an ear infection or treat it before an infection occurs. Decongestants and antihistamines have been used for this purpose, but their effectiveness is now seriously questioned.

## HOME TREATMENT

No home treatment is effective for middle-ear infections. Aspirin or acetaminophen can be given for fever and pain until the antibiotics begin to work. Some parents recommend warm mineral oil or other home preparations to be used as ear drops to try to alleviate the pain. These are questionably helpful and can make it difficult for your physician to examine the eardrum.

## TREATMENT AFTER CONSULTING YOUR PHYSICIAN

As has already been mentioned, antibiotics are the principal treatment for middle-ear infections. There are numerous antibiotics available for your physician. The choice of antibiotic depends on safety, cost, and the type of bacteria that your physician suspects is causing the infection. The most commonly used antibiotic for treatment of middle-ear infections is ampicillin or its close relative, amoxicillin. When taken properly, these antibiotics are effective in over 90% of cases. In approximately 10% of cases, the bacteria causing the infection may be resistant to ampicillin or amoxicillin. If this is the case, your physician will usually change to another antibiotic, either a combination of erythromycin and sulfisoxazole or a combination antibiotic known as trimethoprim/sulfamethoxasole (Bactrim, Septra) or cefaclor (Ceclor). Some physicians will choose to give trimethoprim/sulfamethoxasole as the initial antibiotic for treatment of otitis media because of its effectiveness and because it can be given twice a day instead of three or four times a day. For children who are allergic to ampicillin, erythromycin combined with sulfa is an effective alternative therapy. Cefaclor is an effective but quite expensive antibiotic whose use should be reserved for infections that are resistant to the already mentioned and less expensive antibiotics. Antibiotics are usually continued for ten to fourteen days. Some physicians will treat for a longer period with antibiotics if they feel that the infection has incompletely resolved or that they can eliminate the accumulation of middle-ear fluid. Currently there is no scientific proof that treatment for longer than ten to fourteen days is more effective or that it decreases the chance of fluid accumulating in the middle ear.

Before highly effective antibiotics were available to treat middle-ear infections, physicians treated the infection by making a small incision in the middle eardrum to release the pus and the pressure. This incision, called a *myringotomy*, was quite effective in relieving the pain of middle-ear infections. However, this procedure may cause scarring of the eardrum, and it is not to be recommended as a routine procedure today. In certain situations your physician may need to know if there is still a persistent infection in the middle ear or what the type of bacteria is in the middle-ear fluid that is causing the infection. In this situation, a procedure known as a *tympanocentesis* is performed. Here a sterile needle is placed into the middle ear and the accumulated pus is drawn out and examined. This is not a routine procedure and should be used only when an ear infection has to be diagnosed with absolute certainty.

Some children do not get just two or three infections in their first few years of life but rather are plagued with recurrent ear infections, one frequently following the other with little respite in between. These recurrent ear infections are not only debilitating for the parents and the child but may also cause significant damage to the middle ear. Recurrent ear infections may also cause your toddler's hearing to be significantly compromised for long periods of time during a period of rapid language learning. Some investigators have felt that when this occurs, long-term consequences can be seen in learning problems later in life. This has not been well proven but remains a nagging concern for many physicians and parents.

If your child is afflicted by recurrent ear infections there are two major forms of treatment, one medical and one surgical. Medical treatment consists of continuous administration of antibiotics for a period of six months to one year with the hope of preventing or at least decreasing the frequency of ear infections. It is theorized that six months without infections will allow the middle ear and drainage tubes to repair themselves and enable the natural protective mechanisms of the ear to work. An infection-free six months may also allow your child to get into the summertime when there are less respiratory infections, and if you are lucky to reach the age where incidence of ear infections begins to decrease.

The most commonly used antibiotic for continual treatment of otitis media is sulfisoxazole (Gantrisin). This medicine is given one-half to one teaspoon twice a day for a period of six months to one year. Alternative medicines used for this purpose include ampicillin and trimethoprim/sulfamethoxasole. If your child does not respond to medical treatment it may be necessary to place small tubes between the outer ear and middle ear that allow for equalization of pressure between the outer ear and middle ear and drainage of any accumulated fluid. These tubes are quite effective in preventing ear infections, but unfortunately they fall out, often within a few months. Placement of these tubes also requires that your child be hospitalized and placed under general anesthesia. Because of this we recommend that medical treatment be tried before surgical intervention. Some ear-nose-and-throat specialists also recommend removal of tonsils and/or adenoids for the prevention of recurrent ear infections. This treatment has not been shown to be effective and we do not recommend it for this condition.

### Is the Treatment Working?

The initial antibiotic chosen is usually effective in 90% of ear infections. If your child continues to have fever after forty-eight hours of treatment it is quite possible that the antibiotic has not been working. This may be due to a number of factors:

1. The bacteria in the middle ear is resistant to the antibiotic chosen by your physician.

2. Your child has an ear infection that is not too responsive to the antibiotic although some bacteria are sensitive to it.

3. You may not have been able to give the medicine as frequently as prescribed, or the child may have spit up much of the medicine each time it was given.

If the problem is resistant bacteria, your physician will usually switch to another antibiotic, usually an erythromycin-sulfa combination or trimethoprim/sulfamethoxasole. If your child has one of those ear infections that is not responsive to antibiotics, your physician will usually attempt to change antibiotics but this therapy will not be effective and the middle-ear infection will have to run its own course. If taking the medicine has been a problem for you and your child, let your physician know. This will help to avoid changing to a new and possibly more expensive antibiotic when continued treatment with the same antibiotic would be just as effective.

## OTITIS EXTERNA

### DESCRIPTION

The outer third of the ear canal (from the eardrum to the outside world) has many glands that produce waxy, water-repellent secretion that combines with skin cells that have been shed to form ear wax (cerumen). Ear wax forms a protective coating against the bacteria that normally live in the external ear canal. When the external ear canal becomes excessively wet or dry, the protective effect of the ear wax is diminished, and infection can ensue. Trauma to the ear either from picking and digging or inserting a foreign body can break the protective barrier of the wax and skin and cause infection. Otitis externa can also be caused by other conditions of the skin such as various forms of dermatitis.

### RATIONALE FOR TREATMENT

Treatment for otitis externa is directed at eliminating the infection and reducing the swelling and discomfort that may accompany the infection. If the otitis externa is part of a more generalized skin condition, treatment is directed at the specific condition (see Chapter 26).

### HOME TREATMENT

Mild cases of otitis externa can be treated at home with aluminum acetate solutions (1:40, or half-strength Burrow's solution) that are available without prescription from your pharmacy. This solution can be placed in the ear with an eyedropper three or four times a day, or if there is swelling and pain, applied to a cotton wick in the ear as frequently as possible. If there is no response to this treatment or if there is considerable swelling and pain, you should contact your physician.

One note about prevention. Many parents attempt to remove ear wax from the external canal with a Q-tip or other device, because either they mistake it for dirt or they assume that it interferes with hearing. Rarely does ear wax become impacted in the canal and diminish hearing. If this is the case the wax should be washed out with an ear syringe, and not dug out. Digging out ear wax not only removes the protective coating but also may damage the skin, both of which predispose to infection.

### TREATMENT AFTER CONSULTING YOUR PHYSICIAN

Antibiotic drops can also eradicate infections, although there is no proof they are any more effective than aluminum acetate. Topical preparations often contain the antibiotics colistin and polymyxin as well as neosporin. We do not support the use of neosporin since 2–3% of children may experience an allergic skin reaction with its use. The inflammation of external otitis can be further reduced by solutions (either of aluminum acetate or antibiotics) which are combined with a steroid, usually hydrocortisone. This preparation can be installed three or four times a day or applied frequently with a cotton wick.

## IS THE TREATMENT WORKING?

If the otitis externa is caused by an infection you should see a decrease in symptoms in one to two days. If this does not occur, it may be because

1. you need an anti-inflammatory steroid to reduce the swelling and enable the medication to get to all parts of the external ear canal;

2. the otitis externa may not be caused by infection but instead by another skin condition;

3. you may need a change in antibiotics because of resistant bacteria. This, however, is very unlikely.

If you do not get a response in one to two days, you should contact your physician.

# CHAPTER NINETEEN

# Eye Problems:
## *Conjunctivitis*

## DESCRIPTION

THE CONJUNCTIVA is the clear protective cover that extends over the eyes and on the inner lining of the eyelids. When the conjunctiva is irritated, children experience a wide variety of symptoms. Sometimes the white of the eye will appear pink or red and be recognizable to parents as "pink eye." Other symptoms include itching or burning of the eyes, a sensation of having something caught in the eyes, difficulty looking at light, or a sandy or gritty feeling within the eyes. You may also notice a clear or yellowish discharge draining from the eyes, swelling of the eyelids, or lids being stuck together in the morning.

A variety of conditions can cause conjunctivitis. Every parent has witnessed the redness that follows a vigorous crying episode. Infections, chemical irritants, allergens, trauma, and foreign materials can also cause conjunctivitis.

## RATIONALE FOR TREATMENT

Treatment of conjunctivitis depends on the cause. Each age group has a characteristic set of causes, which will be discussed accordingly. In the newborn period, some infants receive silver nitrate as a preventive measure. Within the first two days of life slightly more than half of these children will experience some form of conjunctival irritation, usually tearing or swelling of the eyelids. However, this should disappear within forty-eight hours and requires no treatment.

Signs of conjunctivitis between the third and fifth day of life may represent conjunctival infection with gonococcus bacteria and should be seen by a physician. Another common infection in the newborn is due to organisms known as chlamydia; this usually occurs by the end of the first week and before the third week of life. These organisms are frequently found in the vaginas of mothers and are a common cause of conjunctivitis in the newborn period. Because the organisms are difficult to eradicate with antibiotic eyedrops, most physicians will elect to treat this infection with a ten-day course of an antibiotic, erythromycin. Treatment with eyedrops requires two to three weeks of treatment, is often unsuccessful, and does not eradicate the chlamydia from the child's nose and mouth, leaving the child susceptible to chlamydia infection of the lungs.

An infant who has tearing in one eye most likely has a plugged tear duct. Better than 90% of blocked tear ducts can be managed satisfactorily by parents with gentle massage with a warm wet cloth over the inner aspect of the eye. Older infants and children most often have conjunctivitis caused by infections, many of which are due to viruses with the rest being caused by bacteria. There is no simple way for you as a parent to tell viral from bacterial infection. Viral infections, however, tend to occur in epidemic outbreaks and are accompanied by other cold symptoms such as a cough. If everyone at school has "pink eye" your child most likely has a viral irritation that will resolve on its own. Herpes is a type of virus that causes serious conjunctival damage. Fortunately, it is extremely rare and usually heralded by eye pain. Any time your child has eye pain, you should see your physician. Bacterial conjunctivitis is quite common, but seldom causes permanent visual problems. Most bacterial conjunctivitis can be treated simply and effectively with antibiotic eyedrops. Bacterial conjunctivitis is sometimes accompanied by ear infections. If your child has both ear pain and conjunctivitis, your physician will most likely treat both problems with antibiotics. Occasionally bacterial conjunctivitis follows the formation of small swellings, called *styes,* on your child's eyelids. A single stye is often not treated. Multiple styes require treatment, usually with antibiotic ointments. If repeated eye infections occur, oral antibiotics and occasionally incision of the styes may be required.

Allergic conjunctivitis usually occurs in preschool and school-age children. It produces itchy eyes and a watery discharge, and it occurs in response to a particular pollen such as ragweed, and may be accompanied by other symptoms such as sneezing or a watery runny nose. Allergic conjunctivitis may cause a pebbly look to the inside lining of your child's lower eyelid. Occasionally, an allergy may be so bad that the conjunctiva will swell, making the eye look mushy in the white portion. Oral antihistamines are often useful in controlling allergic conjunctivitis. Occasionally, eyedrops that constrict or narrow the blood vessels (0.1% naphazoline) may be needed; steroid eyedrops are called for only in the most severe cases. For chronic persistent problems your physicians may recommend special glasses for use during bad pollen seasons.

### HOME TREATMENT

Many things can be done for your child at home. Usually a conjunctivitis is first noticed when the child awakens with eyelids stuck together. Use cotton soaked in warm water to gently melt away the crustings on the lid so that the lids can be parted. If your child complains of a feeling that something is stuck in his or her eye, you can look for small particles by gently retracting the lower lid or by turning the upper lid inside out by rolling it around a cotton swab. Often, however, the feeling that something is stuck in the eye accompanies an abrasion that may have occurred during an injury. When you are suspicious that an injury may have occurred, always see a physician immediately. If you suspect that a chemical has splashed in the eye, rinse the eye out with copious amounts of water. Over-the-counter antihistamines such as diphenhydramine hydrochloride (Benadryl) or chlorpheniramine maleate (chlortrimeton) can be tried for the treatment of allergic conjunctivitis.

*Do not patch your child's eyes.* This will not aid with healing, obscures the progress of the illness, and interferes with vision.

### TREATMENT AFTER CONSULTING YOUR PHYSICIAN

Physician-prescribed therapy is most often directed against infection. Sulfacetamide is one of the most widely prescribed eyedrops. It is available both as an ophthalmic ointment and as a solution, and its reaction rate is fairly low, less than 1%. It is preferred by many physicians for most infections because it has a reaction rate lower than do the other commonly available eyedrops such as gentamicin (10%), and neomycin (15%). Tearing usually washes the solution out fairly quickly. It is therefore important to give this medication as frequently as your physician recommends. However, the ointment is not washed out quite as readily and it does interfere with vision. The ointment is a more acceptable treatment at night. Always be sure to wash your child's lids gently before applying eyedrops, for any pus or crusting may interfere with the action of the sulfacetamide.

In the newborn period, if your physician suspects chlamydia, possible treatments will include either erythromycin eyedrops or oral erythromycin. We prefer the latter because the course of treatment required is ten days instead of two to three weeks, and it appears to be more effective in eradicating the chlamydia.

Occasionally, the infection may spread from the conjunctiva of the eye to involve the skin surrounding the orbit of the eye. This uncommon complication is known as periorbital cellulitis. If it is very early in its course, your physician may elect to treat it with a combination of antibiotics effective against the most common invading bacteria, *Staphylococcus* and *Hemophilus influenzae*. Ampicillin combined with cloxacillin or dicloxacillin is a frequently prescribed combination. Cefaclor has had some success in treatment of this infection, although it is not as good as ampicillin and dicloxicillin in preventing other complications such as meningitis. For allergic conjunctivitis, some physicians may prescribe eyedrops that constrict the blood vessels of the conjunctiva and decrease itching (Vasocon A). Steroid drops have also been used to treat allergic conjunctivitis. This treatment has been reported to cause cataracts (clouding of the lens in the eye) with prolonged administration, and should be used only under the care of a physician. Some physicians will also skin test your child to determine what pollens or allergens are causing the conjunctivitis. This may help your child and avoid potentially allergic substances. We feel, however, that hyposensitization, or allergy shots, are not helpful in the treatment of allergic conjunctivitis.

### IS THE TREATMENT WORKING?

Most infections, viral as well as bacterial, will resolve within three to four days. Chlamydia infections usually take longer to resolve; even if they appear better it is important to continue medication for the fully prescribed treatment period. For most other infections, the treatment should be continued for several days beyond the persistence of symptoms. If your child develops fever following the institution of therapy, or if symptoms become worse, contact your physician. Fever is a sign that the infection may be getting worse. If other symptoms get worse, it is a sign that your child may be allergic to the eyedrops. Recurrent symptoms accompanied by itching and sneezing suggest that allergy is the underlying cause. If your infant continues to have conjunctivitis on one side, this suggests a blocked and possibly infected tear duct. In a very small percentage of infants, massage and antibiotic treatments are insufficient to resolve the problem; usually these children have a web blocking the tear duct that requires gentle surgical probing by an ophthalmologist. Most tear ducts, however, are blocked by cellular debris and require no surgical intervention.

# CHAPTER TWENTY

# Pneumonia

## DESCRIPTION

WHEN CHILDREN are quite ill, especially when they have a bad cold with a cough, many parents will often worry about pneumonia. Pneumonia is a diagnosis that only your physician can make. However, it is seen relatively infrequently, given the number of coughs and fevers children have. You need not worry every time your child has a cough. If your child has a very high temperature (greater than 104°F (40°C) in toddlers, greater than 101°F (38.3°C) in children less than three months of age) or if your child is breathing more rapidly than usual, you should contact your physician.

Although the pronouncement of this diagnosis still produces horrified looks on the faces of most parents we talk with, pneumonia in the 1980s is a fairly benign disease for most children. Pneumonia is an infection that has involved more than the upper airway passage; it involves the lower airway passages as well as some portion of the lung tissue itself. Almost every type of infectious agent can produce pneumonia. Viruses are responsible for most pneumonias. *Mycoplasma*, an organism that is neither a virus nor a bacterium, is also responsible for a considerable number of pneumonias, especially in older children. Bacteria also cause pneumonia, especially three types known as *Hemophilus influenzae, Pneumococcus,* and *Staphylococcus aureus.*

129

RATIONALE FOR TREATMENT

Your physician will diagnose your child's pneumonia based on the physical examination, the chest X-ray, or a combination of the two. Once the diagnosis of pneumonia is made it is often very difficult to determine which infectious agent is responsible. The results of cultures and blood tests take several days to obtain, and physicians will want to begin treatment immediately. Even though most pneumonias are caused by viruses, it is virtually impossible in most cases to reliably predict which pneumonias are viral and which are not. Therefore, most physicians will begin treatment with an antibiotic likely to be most effective against the most likely bacteria causing the infection. Only rarely is hospitalization necessary. This is most often required for younger children, who are also most likely to acquire the most serious type of infection, a *Staphylococcus aureus* infection.

In children less than a year of age *Staphylococcus* can cause pneumonia, and if a chest X-ray reveals a characteristic picture, the child will most likely be hospitalized. Younger children have a preponderance of pneumonias caused by *Hemophilus influenzae*. Antibiotics that eliminate *Hemophilus influenzae* are also effective against the other common bacterial cause of pneumonia, *pneumococcus*. Although it is not truly a bacterium, *Mycoplasma pneumoniae* is a leading cause of pneumonia in older children and adolescents; these organisms will respond to antibacterial agents such as erythromycin and tetracycline. Although these antibiotics do not actually kill the mycoplasma, they cause a marked improvement in the symptoms of the disease.

HOME TREATMENT

There are supportive measures that will be important in treating your child's pneumonia. Acetaminophen or aspirin will provide symptomatic relief of fever. Most children will want to rest, although enforced bedrest will not necessarily hasten resolution of the disease and may precipitate considerable conflict. Vaporizers are of little use and they are effective only in delivering moisture to the very uppermost airway passages.

## TREATMENT WITH MEDICATION

Except in unusual situations where an epidemiologic pattern suggests a viral origin (several children in the family with mild bouts of pneumonia), antibiotics will be prescribed. For younger children, antibiotics effective against *Hemophilus influenzae* such as ampicillin, amoxicillin, or erythromycin-sulfisoxazole combinations will be used. All of these are also effective against *Pneumococcus*. If your physician is convinced that the clinical picture suggests a pneumococcal pneumonia, then a single injection of penicillin or seven to ten days of oral penicillin will be prescribed. If *Mycoplasma* is suspected either erythromycin or tetracycline in older children will be prescribed. Erythromycin-sulfasoxazole combinations are therefore effective against all these pneumonias.

## IS THE TREATMENT WORKING?

After administration of antibiotics is begun for suspected bacterial pneumonia, you should expect to see some improvement by the next day. Viral pneumonias are not affected by antibiotics. If your child is not responding to antibiotics the pneumonia is probably viral. However, if your child appears sick, has a fever over 104°F (40°C), or is breathing rapidly, call your physician. Although the fever may last for a number of days with *Hemophilus pneumoniae* your child should begin looking and feeling better within twenty-four hours or you should contact your physician again. Pneumococcal pneumonias often respond quite dramatically to appropriate antibiotic therapy with disappearance of high fevers often occurring within twenty-four hours. *Mycoplasma pneumoniae* infections seldom have the degree of fever elevation seen with bacterial pneumonias, but characteristically are accompanied by an excessive cough. This symptom should begin to decline within several days.

# CHAPTER TWENTY-ONE

# Vomiting and Diarrhea

## By Ardis Olson, M.D.*

IT IS THE RARE PARENT who does not encounter vomiting and diarrhea at some point in his or her child's life. These are common symptoms that are usually self-limited and not serious. With proper care most cases can be treated at home without a trip to the doctor's office. Occasionally, vomiting and diarrhea can be signs of a more serious illness in your child. In these cases your child will not respond to conventional treatments; he or she will have other symptoms associated with more serious illness. In this chapter we will confine our discussion to the treatment of simple vomiting and/or diarrhea (gastroenteritis) and not attempt to discuss those situations where these symptoms are associated with more serious diseases. If you have any question as to whether your child has a simple case of gastroenteritis or a more serious condition, you should consult your physician.

### DESCRIPTION

*Vomiting* Most parents consider vomiting any spitting up of partially digested food. In young infants "spitting up" is a normal response to a full stomach. This occurs because the muscle at the top of the stomach is not yet strong enough to stop the food from coming up when the stomach contracts. Infants and children will also experience vomiting in response to a virus infection, an allergic response to a new food, or an irritating medicine. In these situations, vomiting

*Practicing pediatrician, Hanover. New Hampshire.

represents the response of an upset stomach to eating and may be an adaptive rejection of substances that cannot be digested or that are too irritating. As we have already mentioned, vomiting is also seen with the obstruction of the digestive tract, and a whole host of other serious illnesses. Until you have lived through a few episodes of vomiting and diarrhea in your child, it can be difficult to determine whether or not your child has a serious illness. A phone consultation with your physician can be helpful in making this decision.

*Diarrhea*   Diarrhea is a sign that your child's gut can no longer properly absorb food and water. This condition can be caused by a virus or bacterial infection, an allergic reaction in the gut, or a particular medicine such as ampicillin. The diarrhea can have different consistencies from watery to semisoft, and can vary from one to twelve or more episodes per day. It is important to consider how different it is from your child's normal bowel habits. A normal pattern for one infant may represent the onset of diarrhea for another.

### RATIONALE FOR TREATMENT

*Vomiting*   When vomiting accompanies a minor illness the goal of treatment, simply put, is to ensure that more liquids stay down than come up, until the illness has run its course. The major danger with vomiting (and diarrhea) is an excessive loss of fluids and important body salts leading to dehydration and a disturbance of the body's chemistry. Treatment is directed at replacing lost fluid and salts in any easy palatable way that will not provoke more vomiting.

*Diarrhea*   What has been said about vomiting can also be said about diarrhea. Treatment is required when there is an excessive loss of water and salt. The goal of treatment is again to replace water and salt in a manner than will not irritate the gut and provoke more diarrhea.

Although it may break your heart as a parent to see your child take only liquids and no "real foods" when being treated for vomiting and/or diarrhea, starvation and malnutrition are not serious concerns for most cases of vomiting and diarrhea. This is why therapy is not directed at replacing lost nutrients in the diet—your child will accomplish this by "overeating" after the illness has ended. In fact, the introduction of fats, proteins, and certain sugars into the diet during an episode of vomiting and/or diarrhea may actually make the symptom worse.

## HOME TREATMENT

Most cases of vomiting and diarrhea can be treated at home.

*Vomiting*   The objective in home treatment of vomiting is to replace the lost water and salts in a manner that is least offensive to a stomach ready to throw back whatever you offer. This can be accomplished by manipulating the kind of liquid given and the manner in which it is given. In choosing a replacement liquid it is important to know that there are certain commonly used liquids that are irritating and difficult to digest. Among these are milk and orange and other citrus juices. Your physician will frequently prescribe a "clear liquid" as a more benign replacement fluid. Some examples of commonly used clear liquids are diluted apple juice (1 part apple juice, 1 part water), flat or defizzed soda pop, dilute liquid gelatin, popsicles, and certain commercial fruit drinks. You should consult with your physician with respect to the choice of a clear liquid. Solid foods and milk are to be avoided in the early treatment of vomiting; they are difficult to digest, are irritating, and frequently will provoke more vomiting.

The manner in which you give clear liquids is also very important. The goal here is to give small amounts of liquids frequently, rather than large amounts less frequently. This ensures that the stomach will not become distended, an event that frequently provokes more vomiting. Many physicians start with 1 to 2 oz every fifteen minutes. If this is successful, the amounts can be advanced and the intervals lengthened. If this is unsuccessful, you may have to give as little as one teaspoon every five to ten minutes. If all regimens fail, you should contact your physician.

*Diarrhea*    Here again the objective is to stay ahead of the game by giving more liquid than is lost through the bowel. With diarrhea, however, generous amounts of fluid may be necessary. For example, a ten-pound infant with diarrhea will require twenty-four to thirty-two ounces of liquid per day; a twenty-pound toddler, forty-eight to sixty-four ounces; and a thirty-pound child, sixty to eighty ounces of fluid per day. The amount of liquid you can "put in" is not limited by gastric irritation and vomiting when your child has only diarrhea.

However, when your child has both vomiting and diarrhea, this task of getting a sufficient amount of fluid into your child can be difficult and time-consuming. Here again the kind of fluid is very important. For the older infant and child, the clear liquids already mentioned are a good place to start. For the smaller infant, for whom the amount and concentration of salts and sugars in the replacement liquid are more critical, special preparations are available without prescription from your pharmacy. The most commonly used formulas are Pedialyte and Lytren. You should consult with your physician as to whether or not to use these special preparations for your child.

There are several medicines available without a prescription for the treatment of diarrhea. The most common active ingredients in these preparations are kaolin (a clay derivative) and pectin (an extract from citrus fruit). These ingredients are designed to thicken the stool. Kaolin and pectin are not harmful; but they do not help the diarrhea. Your child's stools may become thicker, but the frequency and amount of diarrhea and the resulting water loss is unchanged. Because of this, we feel that kaolin and pectin do not have a role to play in the treatment of diarrhea in children. Another type of medicine available without a prescription for the treatment of diarrhea is bismuth salicylate (a metal salt). This compound is found in such medicines as Pepto-Bismol. There is some evidence that Pepto-Bismol is effective in adults in the treatment of certain types of infectious diarrhea acquired when traveling to other countries. It must, however, be given in large doses, up to one bottle per day. We do not know if this treatment works for children with this type of diarrhea. Its effectiveness in other types of diarrhea is also unknown. The use of bismuth salicylate, however, has not been proved safe in young children, and for this reason we do not recommend its routine use in the treatment of diarrhea.

### TREATMENT AFTER CONSULTING YOUR PHYSICIAN

Your physician can assist you in treating your child's vomiting and diarrhea by (1) helping you choose the most appropriate replacement fluid and replacement schedule, (2) evaluating your child for excessive fluid loss (dehydration), (3) and for severe cases, hospitalizing your infant or child for closer evaluation and possible replacement of fluids intravenously.

There are several medicines available by prescription from your physician for the treatment of vomiting and diarrhea. The commonly used medications for treatment of vomiting are promethazine (Phenergan), prochlorpromazine (Compazine), and trimethobenzamide (Tigan). These medicines have been best evaluated in children taking anticancer medicines known to cause vomiting. Although they are probably helpful in this situation, their effectiveness in other types of vomiting is unknown. These medicines, moreover, can have significant side effects. These include sedation, drying of the mouth, disturbances of the nerves and muscles, slurred speech, and mental confusion. Because of these potentially serious side effects, we feel that there is only a limited role for these medications in the treatment of vomiting, and if used, these medications should be used under the close supervision of your physician.

There are several medicines available by prescription that are used to slow down the movement of food through the gut and to decrease the frequency of the diarrhea (Lomotil, diphenoxylate and atropine; Imodium, lopermide; Donnatal and Donnagel, hycosine and atropine). These medicines have been used in adults with noninfectious diarrhea, but they should not be used in children with viral or bacterial diarrhea. These medicines can lead to increased fluid loss in your child; in cases of bacterial diarrhea they may actually make the diarrhea worse. These medicines may also cause dry mouth, excitement, flushing, and increased blood pressure in children in relatively small doses. We feel that there is little or no role for these medicines in the treatment of routine viral and bacterial diarrhea in children.

## Is the Treatment Working?

For most children, careful adherence to a clear liquid diet will result in definite improvement in one to two days. Occasionally, too rapid advancement to a regular diet can lead to a relapse of symptoms. To avoid this problem your physician may recommend advancement to bland, nonmilk, nonfat, constipating foods. A common example of this type of diet is the BRAT diet (B—bananas, R—rice, A—apple sauce and apples, T—toast or dry crackers) with gelatin and other clear liquids being continued for another one to two days. Some physicians will also recommend advancement to a soy formula before restarting a cow's milk formula. This is done to introduce the more easily digestible sucrose sugar (table sugar) before the more difficult to digest lactose sugar (milk sugar). In moderate to severe cases of diarrhea, the gut may take several weeks to completely heal. This means that your child may take two to three weeks to return to normal bowel habits. If your child has not returned to normal after three weeks, or is not continuing to improve, you should contact your physician.

# CHAPTER TWENTY-TWO

# Constipation
By Lucy S. Crain, M.D.*

## DESCRIPTION

CONSTIPATION IS A TERM used to describe hard, dry, and infrequent bowel movements. It is difficult to define constipation in more exact terms, because the normal pattern of bowel movements varies from one individual to the next. It is common for some healthy people, both children and adults, to defecate two or three times a day. Other people, equally healthy, may normally have bowel movements only two or three times a week with no ill effect. The daily bowel movement at a regular time throughout one's life is generally a myth. The most common causes of constipation are inadequate fluid intake, inadequate fiber or bulk in the diet, and inactivity. Constipation may be noted when traveling, caused by changes in diet or routine schedules of meals and/or defecation. Although emotional stress is frequently associated with diarrhea in some people, it may be associated with constipation in others. Children who are "too busy" with schoolwork, playing, or other activities may tend to repeatedly ignore the urge to defecate, thus creating a pattern of chronic constipation. Less commonly, constipation may be a sympton of other organic diseases.

Straining with defecation is the most common complaint associated with constipation. Constipation may be associated with mild abdominal discomfort, often due to gas pains or to

* Associate Clinical Professor of Pediatrics, University of California, San Francisco, California.

ignored defecation urges. Severe abdominal pain is not commonly associated with constipation. Occasionally, a person with appendicitis incorrectly assumes that his or her abdominal pain is due to a need to clean out the bowels. The purgative effect of a laxative on an inflamed appendix may cause the appendix to rupture and cause peritonitis (inflammation of the abdominal cavity or peritoneum). Rarely, severe chronic constipation may result in a fecal impaction, consisting of an accumulation of hard, dry stool in the descending colon and rectum. This condition is almost unheard of in individuals with normal bowel motility (peristalsis), but it can occur in nonambulatory or bedridden, chronically ill individuals if dietary fiber and fluid intake are inadequate.

## RATIONALE FOR TREATMENT

If stools are particularly hard and dry, an individual will usually experience some discomfort in defecation. It is not unusual for infants with hard, dry stools to develop small tears (fissures) of the rectal outlet (anus), resulting in small amounts of bright red blood on the outside of the hard stool. Bleeding in the absence of a visible tear is reason to contact the child's physician.

Relief of such discomfort and straining and prevention of future discomfort are the reasons for treating constipation. However, myths attributing powers to cure or decrease the severity of all sorts of ailments to "a dose of salts" (laxatives) are simply not true.

## HOME TREATMENT

Because there is no such thing as a completely harmless medical laxative, recommended treatments for childhood constipation are readily available at home. Such treatment is related to changing the child's diet to include more bulk and fiber. Constipation is uncommon in breast-fed infants. When it occurs, an infant's stools can be made noticeably looser and straining with defecation decreased by changes in the nursing mother's diet. Such mothers may be advised that including in their diet prunes or prune juice, fresh fruits, and foods that act as natural laxatives for the mother will also have similar action on her nursing infant. Infants who are bottle-fed prepared infant formula generally have somewhat firmer stools than do breast-fed infants. Some prepared formulas produce firmer stools than do others. The stools of both breast- and bottle-fed infants can generally be made softer by the addition of 2 to 4 oz water per day to the infant's diet. Occasionally, the addition of clear corn syrup (e.g., about 1 teaspoon of Karo syrup per 8 oz water) to the supplemental water is required to produce significant softening of the stool.

The diet of older infants (usually four to six months of age or older) can be modified with the addition of strained fruits (e.g., prunes or peaches) or baby cereals in order to produce a softer stool and thus decrease excessive straining with defecation. Similarly, the diet of older children can be modified to change the consistency and moisture content of the stool. Whole-grain or bran cereals or bread, fresh fruits, and leafy green vegetables provide natural fiber and roughage in the diet, increase stool bulk, and stimulate peristalsis. Fruit juices, especially prune juice, stimulate normal peristalsis. The same amount of dietary roughage that produces a stool of desired softness in one child may produce cramping and diarrhea in the next child. Moderation is generally a good rule until the percentage of roughage required by the individual child is determined by reasonable changes in the diet.

### TREATMENT AFTER CONSULTING YOUR PHYSICIAN

Most instances of constipation in children respond to these previously described dietary interventions and do not require medication. The use of suppositories, enemas, and laxatives for children with constipation should be discouraged. If such treatment is considered necessary, it should take place only after a physical examination and under a physician's prescriptive supervision. When such substances are prescribed, it is usually for specific purposes (e.g., emptying of the bowel for an X-ray study or for surgery; temporary use to assist in the establishment of a normal bowel routine). Enemas and glycerin rectal suppositories are used to stimulate the rectum and anus to promote emptying of the last few inches of the bowel. This results in increased peristalsis and additional bowel evacuation. However, use of suppositories or enemas as frequently as once a week may lead to anal irritation and the inability to spontaneously initiate a bowel movement.

If a laxative must be used, stool softeners (docusate) or bulk-forming products may be suggested. Mineral oil (a lubricant or emollient) is an old favorite among laxative advocates. However, its frequent use can lead to interference with absorption of fat-soluble vitamins (e.g., vitamins D, A, K, and E), and it has been implicated as a cause of lipid pneumonia (because of the aspiration of oil into the lungs). Laxatives containing phenolphthalein are bowel stimulants that can produce painful cramping and loss of normal bowel function if used over a long period of time. Salts (saline cathartics) are also bowel stimulants that should especially be avoided by individuals with kidney disease or any problems that might require salt restriction.

### Is the Treatment Working?

Constipation in children is usually a short-term (five to six days) problem caused by stress, dietary changes, or interruptions in the child's usual routine pattern of bowel habits. Reestablishment of routine, removal of stress (e.g., relaxing parents' and child's attitudes about bowel movements and bowel habits), and adding natural bulk and fiber to the child's diet usually result in relief of constipation within three to five days. It is important to remember that some children normally have bowel movements only two or three times per week and that most infants noticeably strain and push with normal defecation. Parents of children who continue to have significant discomfort with hard, dry stools and painful bowel movements after a week's trial of recommended therapy should contact their child's physician for further instructions.

# CHAPTER TWENTY-THREE

# Parasites *(Worms and Protozoa)*

WHEN WE THINK of children and parasites our minds flash to some far corner of the earth where half-starved children with swollen bellies wander aimlessly over a barren landscape. Unfortunately, far-flung corners are not the only places where infestation with parasites is common. The fact is that it is a wormy world: In the United States 20–50% of children at any given time may be infested with roundworm, the protozoa giardia, or pinworms. Fortunately, in most situations the infestation does not cause symptoms and is not harmful. When an infestation causes symptoms that affect your child's well-being, or is highly infectious, treatment becomes necessary. In this chapter we discuss the common parasite infections in the United States (pinworm, roundworm, giardia, and amoeba), when they need treatment, and what are the best medicines.

## PINWORM *(Enterobius vermicularis)*

### DESCRIPTION

Pinworm is perhaps the most common parasite infection affecting children. Up to 25% of children have pinworms at any given time and many of these children will have no symptoms at all. A small percentage, however, will be bothered by mild to intense itching around the anus with the itching classically worse at night.

RATIONALE FOR TREATMENT

When the itching becomes severe, or when a greater than normal amount of scratching is taking place, treatment may be warranted.

HOME TREATMENT

There is no effective home treatment of pinworms. You can make a diagnosis of pinworms by shining a flashlight on the anus at night and looking for small white worms about one-quarter inch in length in the folds of the anus. Your physician can make the diagnosis of pinworms by examining a piece of sticky tape that has been applied to your child's anus for pinworm eggs. This test will occasionally be negative even though the pinworms are there. Because of this fact, many physicians will treat on the basis of symptoms alone.

TREATMENT AFTER CONSULTING YOUR PHYSICIAN

There are two highly effective drugs for the treatment of pinworms, pyrantel pamoate and mebendazole. Both these drugs are 90–100% effective in curing pinworm and can be given in only one dose. Because these drugs are so effective, intensive laundering of bed clothing and underwear is no longer recommended. Occasionally it is necessary to retreat your child in two to three weeks to kill any worms that hatched from eggs ingested at the time of the first treatment. Because pinworm is everywhere in the environment, complete eradication is impossible and reinfection is a common problem.

IS THE TREATMENT WORKING?

If pinworm is the cause of your child's rectal itching, you should notice a marked decrease in the itching in one to two days. If there is no relief of symptoms, you should consider an alternate reason for the symptom.

## ROUNDWORM *(Acaris lumbricoides)*

DESCRIPTION

Roundworm is another extremely common parasite infection (ascariasis) in the United States. Surveys in rural communities in the southern United States show that anywhere from 20% to 64% of children have roundworm infections at any given time. The majority of people with roundworm infection have no symptoms and do not know they are infected unless they pass a worm from the rectum. An occasional child will get discomfort related to the worms in the intestines; this may be abdominal pain, prolonged diarrhea, nausea, vomiting, or when the worms spread from the intestine to the lung, pneumonia.

### RATIONALE FOR TREATMENT

Treatment of roundworm infection is warranted when your child either passes a roundworm or when you go to your physician because your child is symptomatic, and the physician makes the diagnosis of roundworm infection by identifying roundworm eggs in your child's stool.

### HOME TREATMENT

No effective home treatments are available.

### TREATMENT AFTER CONSULTING YOUR PHYSICIAN

Pyrantel pamoate is the drug of choice for the treatment of roundworm infection. It can be administered in one dose with a cure rate of almost 100%.

### IS THE TREATMENT WORKING?

One dose of pyrantel pamoate will effectively kill the roundworm in the gut. However, symptoms caused by the worms may persist for several weeks until healing occurs. Your child may also pass dead worms in his or her bowel movements after treatment; this does not mean that the treatment has failed. Some children will occasionally have an allergic reaction to the breakdown products of the dead worm and will feel worse after treatment. If this occurs, you should consult your physician.

### AMOEBA *(Entamoeba histolytica)*

### DESCRIPTION

Infection with amoeba (amebiasis) is a common health problem affecting anywhere from 1% to 10% of children in the United States. The majority of children infected with amoeba will not have symptoms or will have vague symptoms such as stomachache, belching, nausea, or fullness of the stomach. A certain percentage of children, however, will develop a severe inflammation of the gut characterized by painful abdominal cramps and bloody diarrhea. An even smaller percentage of children will develop infection outside the gut—in the liver, in the sac around the heart, or even in the brain, where infections can lead to serious complications.

## RATIONALE FOR TREATMENT

Because of the potential for serious complication all cases of amebiasis should be treated. It is most likely, however, that your child would be treated only if he or she has become symptomatic, or has come in close contact with a known carrier. Diagnosis is usually made by examination of the stool. Occasionally direct examination of the gut through a special scope (proctosigmoidoscope) or blood tests may be necessary. It is important to make the diagnosis before treating to make sure that you are not missing another treatable condition and not to needlessly expose your child to potentially (albeit only a small potential) harmful medicines.

## TREATMENT AFTER CONSULTING YOUR PHYSICIAN

Several medicines are available for the treatment of amoeba. For the child that is asymptomatic the most commonly used drugs are metronidazole (Flagyl) or iodoquinol (Yodoxin). If your child is symptomatic with diarrhea or other major symptoms the most commonly used drugs are metronidazole, tetracycline (for children eight years or older) plus iodoquinol or dihydroemetine plus iodoquinol. These drugs vary in their efficacy and side effects, with no one preparation being the best choice for all situations. The choice of antibiotic(s) should be discussed with your physician.

## IS THE TREATMENT WORKING?

When the amoeba infection has been confined to the gut,

one or a combination of these previously mentioned antibiotics will cure the infection in over 90% of cases. Because tissue invasion of the gut can cause significant damage to the lining of the gut, healing (and relief of symptoms) may take several weeks to occur. You should, however, expect some relief within one to two days.

## GIARDIA *(Giardia lamblia)*

### DESCRIPTION

Giardia is the most common protozoan parasite affecting children. Surveys of children in the United States have shown that up to 20% can harbor giardia in their stools at any given time. Most of these children will have no symptoms and will eliminate the giardia without the benefit of antibiotics. Some children will develop diarrhea and abdominal cramps, and will lose weight.

### RATIONALE FOR TREATMENT

Any child with significant symptoms from giardia should be treated with antibiotics because of the possibility of prolonged discomfort and malnutrition from the diarrhea and cramps. Because giardia can be passed from child to child, children without symptoms should be treated if they come into contact with other children.

### HOME TREATMENT

There is no effective home treatment. Symptomatic relief for diarrhea is discussed in Chapter 21.

### TREATMENT WITH MEDICATION

The first problem your physician has in treating giardiasis is making the diagnosis. It can take repeated examination of your child's stool (up to six) to find the giardia. Occasionally your physican will have to aspirate and examine the contents of the gut to find the organism. Again, it is important for your physician to make the diagnosis before treatment so that he or she does not overlook another potentially serious illness and expose your child unnecessarily to the possible side effects of the required antibiotics.

There are two effective (70–95% cure rates) antibiotics used for the treatment of giardia, quinacrine (Atabrine) and metronidazole (Flagyl). Both these medicines have potential side effects, and the choice of antibiotic should be discussed with your physician.

### Is the Treatment Working?

Treatment with the appropriate antibiotic kills the giardia rapidly and effectively. You should see an improvement in symptoms within two to three days. Again, some symptoms may persist for several weeks, until the gut has completely healed. Occasionally treatment will cure your child of symptoms, but not completely eliminate the giardia. Your physician should check the stool after treatment to make sure the giardia has been eliminated. If it still persists, retreatment or change of medicine and retreatment may be necessary.

## PARASITES AND THE FAMILY

Finally it is important to note that parasite infections in children frequently involve other members of the family even if these other family members have no symptoms. Because of this you should discuss with your physician the need for checking other members of the family and treating them for the parasite when necessary.

# CHAPTER TWENTY-FOUR

# Urinary Tract Infections

## DESCRIPTION

URINARY TRACT INFECTION (cystitis, bladder infections, kidney infections, pyelonephritis) are among the most common infections affecting children. The urinary tract consists of the kidney, ureter, bladder, and urethra (see illustration). Although the urinary tract is open to the outside world through the urethra, it is able to protect itself from the germs or bacteria that reside on children's bottoms and that can potentially cause infection. In some children, however, bacteria grow on the skin around the opening of the urethra that are different from normal skin bacteria and that have a much greater potential of causing infection. This process occurs when the bacteria ascend from the opening of the urethra to the bladder, where they find a warm, wet world in which they readily grow and cause infection.

Once the bacteria are in the bladder, they may also ascend from the bladder to the kidneys by a process known as reflux. An infection of just the bladder is called *cystitis,* and an infection that involves the kidney is called *pyelonephritis.*

## RATIONALE FOR TREATMENT

When infection involves just the bladder, there may be painful symptoms but hardly ever any permanent damage to the urinary tract. However, if the infection spreads to the kidney and is not properly treated, significant damage can occur to that kidney in a matter of months. The most important issue,

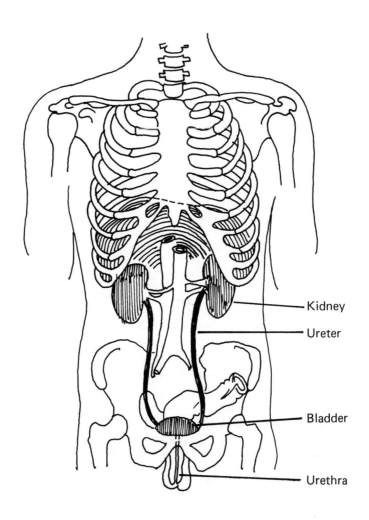

Kidney

Ureter

Bladder

Urethra

therefore, in treating the urinary tract infection is to kill the bacteria in the urinary tract and make sure that that bacteria do not ascend to cause reinfection in the bladder or kidney. The treatment prescribed for the urinary tract infection will depend on whether the infection is confined to the bladder or whether it has spread to the kidney.

## HOME TREATMENT

The major purpose of home treatment is to provide relief of the symptoms until the proper antibacterial medicine can be prescribed. Such treatments as making the urine acid with cranberry juice or some other acid foodstuff, or attempting to flush out the infection by taking increased amounts of fluids, may help alleviate some of the symptoms but they will not treat or prevent a urinary tract infection.

For symptomatic relief, acetaminophen (Tylenol, Datril, Liquiprin) can provide some relief of the pain that can occur with a urinary tract infection. Drinking increased amounts of fluid can also ease the urgency of urination. The doctor may also prescribe a medicine that is available for the treatment of pain associated with urinary tract infection. This medicine, called phenazopyridine hydrochloride (Pyridium), comes only in pill form and in doses designed primarily for older children. It is variably effective in diminishing pain, but in some children it may be quite effective. If your child has recurrent urinary tract infections, it may be useful to keep this medicine at home to provide symptomatic relief until the antibiotic begins to work. When taking this medicine, it is important to remember that one of its major side effects is that it turns your urine an orange color.

Finally, it is important to remember that the taking of antibiotics at home before your physician has been consulted or before a culture of the urine has been taken can compromise your physician's ability to diagnose and treat the infection.

## TREATMENT AFTER CONSULTING YOUR PHYSICIAN

The major objective in treating the urinary tract infection is to eliminate the infection by killing the bacteria. This will allow the urinary tract to heal and the symptoms to subside. To kill the bacteria, antibiotic medicines are needed. There are three major antibiotics used to treat urinary tract infections, chosen because they achieve high concentrations in urine, have extensive bacterial killing power, and have minimal serious side effects. The most commonly prescribed antibiotic for treatment of urinary tract infection is sulfisoxazole (Gantrisin). This medicine can be given in a liquid or pill form, four times a day for a period of ten days. Some physicians have been giving the medicine for a short period of time and in some cases in a single dose. These shorter courses of treatment have not been proven effective in children and as such should be discussed with your physician before they are used. The other commonly prescribed medicines are ampicillin and its close relative, amoxicillin. These medicines are given in liquid or pill form, three or four times a day. Again, there has been some evidence showing that for most urinary tract infections one dose of the medicine (this is particularly true for amoxicillin) may be sufficient. This treatment has only been evaluated in a few studies involving children and again should be discussed with your physician. Trimethoprim/sulfamethoxazole (Bactrim, Septra) has been primarily used for prevention of urinary tract infections, but it can be used also for the treatment of an ongoing infection. This medicine has the advantage that it can be given as a liquid or a pill only twice a day. Single-dose treatment has also been successful with this medication, but again, however, because of its experimental nature, you should discuss this treatment with your physician.

There are a host of additional antibiotics that are capable of treating urinary tract infections. These are not regularly employed because of either excessive cost or serious side effects. However, an additional antibiotic may have to be used in certain situations when the bacteria involved is resistant to one of these mentioned drugs. If the urinary tract infection involves the kidneys (pyelonephritis), a more intensive treatment regimen may be prescribed. This can involve longer treatment (single-dose treatments are probably not effective in pyelonephritis) with higher doses of medicine. In some cases, your physician may even hospitalize your child to give the medications intravenously.

For children with urinary tract infections, and particularly for school-age girls with urinary tract infections, recurrence of that infection is the rule rather than the exception. In fact, if your child has had one urinary tract infection, he or she has an 80% chance that the infection will recur. As already mentioned, if these infections are confined primarily to the bladder there is almost never any serious permanent damage to the urinary tract. However, if the infection has involved the kidney, serious damage can ensue from recurrent infections. Prevention of recurrent urinary tract infections can be achieved through the continuous administration of antibiotics. If your child's urinary tract infections have been confined to the bladder, your physician may wish to see if the condition will spontaneously resolve before deciding to give antibiotics. However, if frequent urinary tract infections do occur with their concomitant painful symptoms and absence from school, antibiotics may be given to prevent further infections. If your child, however, has as little as one infection involving the kidney, antibiotics may be necessary to prevent further infection and insure that no damage occurs to the kidneys. Antibiotics used to prevent urinary tract infections are usually given a six-months to one-year trial period. After the trial period is finished, your child will be taken off antibiotics and the urine checked periodically to make sure the infection has not recurred. If the infection does recur, it may be necessary to start the antibiotics again.

Two antibiotics are commonly used for prevention of infection. Trimethoprim/sulfamethoxazole is the most commonly prescribed medicine for this purpose. It can be given as a liquid or a pill and is effective in a low dose given every other day. It is the preferred medicine for prevention because of its effectiveness in eliminating the problem bacteria on the skin surrounding the opening of the urethra, and because it can be given in a low dose infrequently. Nitrofurantoin (Furadantin, Macrodantin) has also been prescribed for the prevention of urinary tract infections. This medicine can again be given as a liquid or a pill on a daily basis, but it is less desirable than trimethoprim/sulfamethoxazole because of its higher incidence of minor side effects (stomach upset) and serious side effects (lung problems).

### IS THE TREATMENT WORKING?

The bacteria in the urinary tract may be killed with as little as one dose of medicine. However, it may take one to two days for the swelling and inflammation caused by that infection to decrease and consequently for the worst of the symptoms to diminish. It is not unusual to have some minor symptoms persist for several days. You should, however, expect a major improvement in symptoms in twenty-four to forty-eight hours. If this does not occur, the medicine may not be working and you should contact your physician. The only way you can be absolutely sure that the medicine has worked is for your doctor to take a sample of urine after the treatment is finished to see if any bacteria remain. You should expect your physician to re-culture your child's urine after the treatment has been completed. When antibiotics are being given to prevent urinary tract infections, you should expect no recurrence of symptoms. If symptoms do recur, you should call your physician immediately and a culture of the urine should be taken. Unfortunately, urinary tract infections can recur without symptoms and still be damaging to the kidney. Because of this, your physician should check your child's urine at regular intervals to ensure that the medicine is indeed preventing the growth of bacteria in the urinary tract.

# CHAPTER TWENTY-FIVE

# Bedwetting

## DESCRIPTION

BEDWETTING (nocturnal enuresis) has been a problem to parents for quite some time. Reference to enuresis was made as long ago as 1550 B.C. in the Ebers papyrus; and it is questionable if much has been done to resolve this symptom in the intervening years.

In this chapter, we will confine our discussion to enuresis that occurs at night (nocturnal enuresis). Enuresis occuring during the day is a less common and more complex event and demands a different approach. If your child has daytime wetting, you should consult your physician.

The first problem with bedwetting is, when is it a problem? In tropical cultures, where clothes are scant and the sun is warm, enuresis is not considered a problem in children. Certain Western European societies, however, unrealistically expect children to be toilet trained by the age of six months. In order for you, as a parent, to know when to consider bedwetting abnormal (bedwetting can be a normal developmental phenomenon, and still be a problem) it is essential to understand how common bedwetting is in children at various ages:

| Age *(years)* | % of Children with Nocturnal Enuresis |
|---|---|
| 4 | *12–28%* |
| 6 | *10–13* |
| 8 | *7–10* |
| 10 | *3–5* |
| 12 | *2–3* |
| 18 | *2* |

You can see that bedwetting is not uncommon until the age of twelve years or older. This information has had important implications for you as a parent: (1) Any problem that is this common at younger ages and that becomes increasingly rare at older ages most likely reflects the ongoing process of normal neuromuscular development rather than some serious illness or family psychopathology. Less than 5% of children with bedwetting have a medical problem. (2) No matter what you do (or preferably do not do) the odds are in your favor that bedwetting will go away with time.

Bedwetting, however, can be a problem even when it is not "abnormal." For a busy family, the prospect of washing and changing sheets nightly can be the straw that breaks the camel's back. Bedwetting may also prevent the older child from participating in slumber parties, going to overnight camp, or going on camping trips. If enuresis causes considerable strife in your family, or dysfunction in your child, you may wish to consider more aggressive treatment of the symptom than waiting until he or she "outgrows" it.

## RATIONALE FOR TREATMENT

When considering treatment strategies for bedwetting it is important to separate children with medical and psychosocial causes for enuresis from those for whom it is a manifestation of develpmental delay. Because up to 5% of children with bedwetting may have a medical problem, it is important that you check with your physician. In general, a physical examination, and an examination of the urine under a microscope are sufficient evaluation for possible medical causes. The routine use of X-rays of the urinary tract, or examination of the bladder through a tube or scope (endoscopy) is not called for, and can be harmful. Only rarely does a child need these procedures. If a medical cause is found (the most common of these is urinary tract infection), it should be appropriately treated. It should be noted, however, that treatment of the medical condition may not eliminate bedwetting.

Bedwetting can also be a manifestation of emotional problems in your child. If you suspect that this might be the case, you should work with your physician to sort out the developmental, psychological, and medical components of the problem and to determine the appropriate treatment. If the bedwetting is a developmental phenomenon that either has gone too long for your liking or is causing significant problems in your family, you can try some of the treatments described in the following section. In general, these treatments cannot enhance maturation of the muscles and nerves in the bladder that control urination. They can, however, reinforce certain behaviors and habits in your child to increase the probability of staying dry at night, or change the neuromuscular action of the bladder such that your child can more effectively "hold onto" urine. Because none of these treatments deals with the functional problem of maturational delay, none of them is completely successful, and many have significant relapse rates. You should not expect complete elimination of bedwetting, which usually comes only with time.

## HOME TREATMENT

The first, and easiest, way to treat bedwetting at home is to help your child avoid the symptom altogether. This can be accomplished by first observing at what time of night your child wets his or her bed. Once this is done, purchase your child an alarm clock and teach your child to set the alarm at the time that will allow awakening before the enuresis occurs. This method does not work well if the time of bedwetting is variable, or if the child is such a deep sleeper that he or she does not respond to the alarm clock (you, on the other hand, will be invariably awakened by the alarm clock). Do not expect perfect results. Start with a reasonable goal such as decreasing bedwetting by one or two times a week so that your child does not feel that he or she has failed. Eventually you may decrease the number of nights per week that you set the alarm, in the hope that you have trained your child to the point when he or she will automatically awaken before bedwetting occurs. There have not been scientific studies to evaluate the effectiveness of this method. In our opinion, it is reasonably effective in up to 50% of children. Because it is easy and because it gives the child a sense of control, we feel that it is a good method to try first. One provision with this method: make sure that your child does not become fatigued from the night waking. Also, do not set the alarm more than two times a night, for this will be disruptive to your child's sleep.

Another safe and easy method for controlling bedwetting is bladder exercises. Here the child, on feeling the urge to urinate, is asked to hold his or her urine for a set period of time before urinating. This time period is then gradually increased with the hope of increasing bladder capacity and the child's ability to hold his or her urine until a toilet can be reached. This method has been somewhat successful, with one study showing success in up to one-third of the children.

Another commonly employed method of training the body to awaken before enuresis occurs is the urine-alarm method. Basically, the apparatus consists of a urine-sensitive pad that triggers an alarm (usually a bell) that awakens the child who then voluntarily stops urinating and holds the urine until a toilet can be reached. This method has been well studied in bedwetting children. Briefly summarized, the results of these studies show that with an average treatment of five weeks, 75% of patients will have no, or decreased episodes of, enuresis. Also of importance is the fact that 41% of these children will relapse after treatment. This relapse can be treated again by another course with the urine-alarm method. The advantage of this method is that it has been thoroughly evaluated and is probably the most effective method of treating enuresis over the short term. Long-term evaluation has not been done, but with such a high relapse rate it is doubtful that this method is more effective after a period of two years than no treatment at all. The disadvantage of this method is that it does cost money (the apparatus costs thirty to forty dollars), and it may be psychologically traumatic to your child. These disadvantages should be carefully weighed against the advantages of short-term improvement of the bedwetter.

Another method that has been advocated by health professionals for bedwetting is water deprivation before bedtime. Water deprivation, or allowing no liquid intake in your child between the end of dinner and bedtime, has not been shown to be effective in the treatment of bedwetting. Moreover, your child may interpret water deprivation as a punishment for a condition that is not his or her fault, and out of his or her voluntary control. This can lead to a feeling of guilt, and a loss of self-esteem.

### TREATMENT AFTER CONSULTING YOUR PHYSICIAN

When the previously mentioned methods have failed, and bedwetting is still causing considerable problems, you may wish to consider drug treatment with imipramine. Although imipramine was initially developed as an antidepressant for adults, it also acts on the bladder muscle, and affects the sleep cycles. It is these latter two actions, and not its antidepressant effect, that make it useful in treating bedwetting. Imipramine is given one-half hour before bedtime; the dose is increased nightly until the desired effect is achieved or until a maximum dose, ranging from 40 mg in the five-to-six-year-old to 75 mg in the ten-to-twelve-year old, is reached. Imipramine has been reasonably successful in the short-term treatment of enuresis, with scientific studies showing success in up to 50% of children. The relapse rate is high, and re-treatment is frequently needed. Optimal effects are usually achieved in one to two weeks. If your child has not had any success at the maximum dose for this time peroid, the medicine should be discontinued. Once the desired effect has been achieved, the medicine should be continued for two to three months and then gradually withdrawn. Common side effets include drowsiness, dryness of the mouth, restlessness, sleep disturbances, and mood changes. More importantly, imipramine is an extremely toxic drug with as little as 500 mg being lethal if ingested by a toddler. Because of this, we recommend extreme caution where toddlers or older infants are present.

## IS THE TREATMENT WORKING?

With any of these treatments complete elimination of enuresis over a short period of time is unlikely. Establish a reasonable goal with your child, initially start conservatively—for example, to be dry one or two nights per week—and gradually increase the number of dry days per week. Anticipate relapses after the treatment modality is withdrawn. Let your child know that these may occur, and that they do not mean that he or she has failed. If a treatment has not been effective over a given period of time (usually one to two months), discard it. Remember, your child may not respond, or may only partially respond, to these treatments. To push treatment further in this situation can be frustrating and psychologically damaging to your child. Remember, over the long run, enuresis is one problem your child will probably outgrow.

# CHAPTER TWENTY-SIX

# Skin Problems

THE SKIN IS the largest organ in the body, and certainly the most visible. Problems affecting the skin seem to cry out for attention; it is hard not to do something for those spots all over your child's body. Unfortunately, "doing something" for your child's skin problems may cause more difficulties than doing nothing at all. In this section, we hope to help with this dilemma by identifying those conditions for which home treatment (or no treatment) is the best alternative, and those conditions that require a trip to the physician for more intensive medical care. This chapter will be divided into six parts: infections of the skin, infestations, diaper rashes, allergic reactions of the skin, acne, seborrheic dermatitis (cradle cap, dandruff), eczema (atopic dermatitis), and sunburn.

# Infections

Infections of the skin can be divided into two categories: those conditions in which the skin is part of a more widespread infection, and those conditions in which the infection primarily affects the skin. We will spend most of our time on the latter conditions because it is here that we can accomplish the most therapeutically. First, however, a few words about infections that affect the whole body including the skin.

161

Common examples of this type of infection are most often encountered when children are growing up: measles, German measles (rubella), and chicken pox. Because of recent advances in immunization against measles and rubella, it is unusual to see these infections today. It is still common, however, to see "measley" rashes caused by organisms other than measles. Some common examples of this are roseola, a red rash all over the body associated with high fever in young children; Fifth's disease, another red rash primarily on the arms and legs; and what your physician may call non-specific viral infections. Because the rash in these illnesses is caused by a viral illness affecting the whole body, there is little that can be applied directly to the skin that will affect the course of the rash. You may be able to provide symptomatic relief for itchiness, but you cannot cure or hasten the elimination of the rash in this situation (we will discuss treatment of itchy rashes in the section on Allergic Conditions of the Skin). An attempt to treat these rashes with a wide variety of salves or creams may induce an allergic reaction and make things worse. This is one situation when waiting and watching is usually the best course of action.

There are, however, some exceptions to this rule that should be noted. Certain infections of the body caused by bacteria produce a rash as their most notable symptom and need treatment with an antibiotic to prevent complications. The most common example of this is scarlet fever, an infection caused by the streptococcus bacterium and treated with penicillin to prevent rheumatic fever. There are numerous other examples of infections with skin rashes that demand treatment with antibiotics. In general, if your child has one of these infections he or she will be sufficiently sick that you will seek the help of your physician in determining the most appropriate treatment.

Infections that primarily affect the skin can be mild illnesses that are easily treated at home or serious infections requiring hospitalization and intravenous antibiotics. In general, the more serious infections are caused by bacteria and the more minor infections by viruses and funguses. We will start by discussing bacterial infections and then move on to virus and fungus infections of the skin.

# IMPETIGO

## DESCRIPTION

The most common bacterial infection of the skin, and the best known, is impetigo. Impetigo is caused when bacteria (group A streptococci) that are normally found on the skin of healthy children manage to break through the protective barrier of the skin surface and establish an infection. This breakdown in the normal protective mechanisms of the skin may come from a small scratch or an abrasion, from a mosquito bite, or from no discernible cause at all.

## RATIONALE FOR TREATMENT

In almost all cases, this is a minor infection that is not serious; it may, however, as one of its complications cause an inflammatory reaction in the kidney called glomerulonephritis. This complication is rare and cannot be prevented with antibiotics. Because impetigo is infectious to other children and because it frequently continues to spread without treatment, most cases will require treatment.

## HOME TREATMENT

Much of what has been written on the home treatment of impetigo has focused on the importance of hygiene for your child. Although reasonable hygiene is encouraged for all children, the fact that your child has impetigo does not mean that he or she is the hygienic equivalent of a street urchin from a Dickens novel. You cannot be assured that by bathing your child twice a day and boiling his or her clothes and bedding in antiseptics you will necessarily prevent impetigo. Although good hygiene is important to the health of your child, extraordinary hygienic measures should not be a part of the home treatment of impetigo.

In the past, home treatment of impetigo frequently involved peeling off the crust of the sore, exposing the sore to the sun, or dabbing an antibiotic powder or ointment onto the skin. Some physicians also recommended soaking sores, removing the crust, and then applying an antibiotic ointment to the base of the sore. Although they may be partially effective in the treatment of impetigo, these measures may also be painful and traumatic to your child. Today with the advent of highly effective antibiotics, we feel that these measures are not necessary and that the treatment is more easily and effectively accomplished with oral antibiotic medicines.

### TREATMENT AFTER CONSULTING YOUR PHYSICIAN

Once the diagnosis of impetigo has been made, your physician will most likely prescribe an oral antibiotic for your child. Some physicians use topical (applied to the sore itself) antibiotic ointments or soap and water to treat small isolated spots of impetigo. However, topical treatment is not as effective as oral treatment and should not be used when there is more than one area involved, when there is a large area of involvement, or when the face is involved. The most common antibiotics used to treat impetigo are penicillin and erythromycin, chosen because they are the safest antibiotics with respect to side effects, and are the least expensive. If you and your physician decide on penicillin, you can give it as either a liquid or a pill four times a day for ten days, or as a single injection. The injection has the obvious advantage of not having to give the medicine four times a day for ten days, but has the disadvantage of being painful and having a higher incidence of serious allergic reaction. Erythromycin may also be given as a liquid or a pill four times a day for ten days, but it is not available as an injection. Some types of impetigo, particularly those types characterized by large, pus-filled blisters, may be caused by the staphylococcus bacterium. If this is the case, your physician will most likely choose cloxacillin, dicloxacillin, or erythromycin as the antibiotic of choice. All of these must be given orally, four times a day for ten days.

### IS THE TREATMENT WORKING?

If the antibiotic is working, the spots of impetigo should

cease from spreading. The spots that exist should begin to dry up within forty-eight hours. If the spots of impetigo do not stop spreading or do not dry up within forty-eight hours, you should consult your physician. Unfortunately, your child will not build up any resistance to impetigo by having had a prior infection. Because of this, your child may catch impetigo again after the treatment is over. This is particularly true if your child is in a classroom or day-care setting where impetigo is easily spread. It is important that you do not confuse reinfection with impetigo with treatment failure.

## CELLULITIS

### DESCRIPTION

Cellulitis is a more serious infection of the skin characterized by a diffuse infection of the underlying tissue as well as of the skin surface. It is caused by a Staphylococcus, Streptococcus, or Hemophilus bacterium. These infections arise from the introduction of the bacteria into a cut or an abrasion or the spread of a blood-borne infection into the skin.

### RATIONALE FOR TREATMENT

Cellulitis has the potential of spreading quickly and causing serious illness. It demands immediate treatment with antibiotics and a close follow-up, often every day, to ensure that the antibiotics are working.

### HOME TREATMENT

There is no adequate home treatment of cellulitis. Although elevation of the involved area and hot soaks to that area may be helpful, they are not sufficient to stop the infection. If you suspect a cellulitis infection, you should contact your physician immediately.

### TREATMENT AFTER CONSULTING YOUR PHYSICIAN

If the cellulitis is well localized to one part of the skin and if there is no evidence that it is part of a blood-borne infection, your physician will most likely treat it with antibiotics given by mouth. The ones most commonly employed are penicillin, cloxacillin, dicloxacillin, ampicillin, and cefaclor. These antibiotics are available in pill or liquid form and are given four times a day for a minimum period of ten days. If the area involved is more extensive, or if there is evidence of blood-borne infection, intravenous therapy with antibiotics may be necessary. In this case, different antibiotics are used and the choice of antibiotics and their side effects should be discussed with your physician.

### Is the Treatment Working?

You will know that the antibiotics are working if the cellulitis stops spreading in six to twelve hours and the area of redness becomes smaller within twenty-four to forty-eight hours. Any accompanying symptoms such as fever or "feeling sick" should disappear within twenty-four hours. If these signs fail to occur, you should notify your physician immediately.

# BOILS OR FURUNCLES

### Description

Boils or furuncles are another common bacterial infection of the skin. A boil is a localized infection of the skin surrounding the opening of a hair or the hair follicle. The infection is usually localized to the hair follicle, or if it does spread, it spreads very slowly.

### Rationale for Treatment

Most furuncles will resolve on their own without any treatment. Occasionally, a furuncle will become large and painful or will spread beyond the hair follicle; if this occurs, treatment is required.

### Home Treatment

Because this is an infection that is localized to the hair follicle, it responds readily to hot soaks. These should be applied with a towel or compress three to four times a day for a period of twenty minutes each.

### TREATMENT AFTER CONSULTING YOUR PHYSICIAN

Should the furuncle continue to grow in size and become more painful despite the treatment with hot soaks, antibiotics may be required. Here the antibiotics of choice must be active against the Staphylococcus bacterium; the most commonly used ones are dicloxacillin, cloxacillin, and erythromycin.

### IS THE TREATMENT WORKING?

You will know that the hot soaks are working if the boil reduces in size and redness, or if the pus within the boil comes to a head and drains. If antibiotics are used, the boil will frequently not come to a head and drain pus, but you should see some decrease in the size of the boil, the redness, and the amount of pain within forty-eight hours.

## VIRAL INFECTIONS OF THE SKIN: WARTS

### DESCRIPTION

The most common viral infection affecting the skin is the wart. Warts can take anywhere from one to six months to develop, and up to 65% of them will disappear spontaneously within two years.

### RATIONALE FOR TREATMENT

Because the majority of warts disappear on their own, it is often best to watch and wait, rather than to treat them. Overzealous efforts to eradicate warts are not only painful but can lead to permanent scarring. One should consider treating a wart when it becomes painful and interferes with function, or when its appearance becomes unsightly.

### HOME TREATMENT

Most common warts found on the hands of children, and occasionally on the legs, can be effectively treated with over-the-counter preparations from your drug store. Warts on the face, and warts located near nails or the genitals, may be difficult to treat and can have a high potential for scarring.

These warts should be treated in consultation with your physician. For common warts, the use of nonprescription drugs containing salicylic acid and lactic acid (Duofilm) is an effective form of treatment in 60–80% of patients. When treating warts with these preparations, first wash the area thoroughly with soap and water, then rub the surface of the wart gently with a mild abrasive, such as an emery board or pumice stone. Apply the medicine to the wart with a sharp pointed stick, such as a match stick or an orange stick. Allow the medicine to dry and repeat this each night. If the area becomes red or tender, stop the therapy until these symptoms disappear and then start again. If the redness appears again, consult your physician for alternative therapies. Treatment of warts with these preparations is a slow and steady process; complete disappearance of the wart may take up to twelve weeks.

Warts on the bottom of the feet, or plantar warts, are so difficult to eliminate that often the best treatment may be no therapy or a nonaggressive therapy such as flattening the wart with a pumice stone or a callous file. If, however, the wart is painful or is rapidly growing more extensive treatment may be necessary. Therapy with the above described salicylic and lactic acid preparation can be effective in the treatment of these warts. If you do decide to treat plantar warts with these preparations, first rub the surface of the wart with a pumice stone or emery board and soak the foot in hot water or a bath for at least five minutes. Then apply a drop of the medicine to the wart and allow it to dry. After the wart is dry, apply a piece of adhesive tape; repeat this therapy nightly. If soreness occurs, stop the treatment and restart it after it subsides. Again, remember treatment of plantar warts is a slow process and it may take twelve weeks or more for the wart to disappear.

## TREATMENT WITH MEDICATION

There are several wart treatments available only through your physician. The most commonly used of these treatments is liquid nitrogen. This therapy is quick and very effective. For common warts on the hands or legs, frequently only three treatments at weekly intervals are required, when home treatment may require twelve weeks. The disadvantages of liquid nitrogen therapy are that it is painful during its application (this pain lasts approximately ten to fifteen seconds) and it requires a trip to the doctor's office to receive the treatment. Electrosurgery is another method available to your physician for the treatment of warts. Here a high-voltge, low-amperage current is applied directly to the wart, causing its destruction. The advantage of this therapy is again that it is quick and may shorten the course of treatment; but like liquid nitrogen it is painful during application. Moreover, electrosurgery can leave small light-colored scars on the skin. In general, we do not recommend the use of liquid nitrogen or electrosurgery to treat warts in children. This is because the treatments are painful and potentially traumatic to your child. If short-term pain tolerance is not a problem for your child, however, liquid nitrogen is a quick and effective form of therapy. It is also possible for your physician to prescribe a prescription medicine for the treatment of warts, cantheridin (Cantharone), a cell poison that causes destruction and blister formation around the wart.

We recommend a trip to the physician when (1) home treatment has failed, (2) your child's warts are on the face, or (3) when you want to remove the wart quickly.

## Is the Treatment Working?

Treatment of warts is often only partially successful. At any time during the therapy it is possible to reinfect the nearby skin with wart virus and produce new warts. Moreover, there is no positive way to be sure with any of the previously described treatments that all the virus has been killed. Recurrence after treatment is not uncommon, and prevention is difficult to accomplish.

In treating a wart with a salicylic acid/lactic acid preparation, you should notice a scaling and peeling of the wart that gradually leads to a disappearance of the wart over a period of six to twelve weeks. If there is no decrease in the size of the wart by six weeks or disappearance of the wart by twelve weeks, the treatment is not working and your physician should be consulted. When your child is treated with liquid nitrogen therapy, you will notice a reaction to the liquid nitrogen ranging from redness and scaling to a full-blown blister that can be filled with blood. This represents a killing of the wart and is not a sign of infection. When you return to your physician, he or she will scrape away the dead skin and will treat again with liquid nitrogen. This will be repeated until the wart has disappeared. You should expect the wart to have disappeared after three to four treatments with liquid nitrogen. The exceptions to this are plantar warts, which may take up to twelve weeks to treat.

## FUNGUS INFECTIONS OF THE SKIN

### DESCRIPTION

Fungus infections are a common problem afflicting children. When the infection is confined to the skin, it is commonly called ringworm (this name comes from the ringlike appearance of the skin infection and not from the presence of any worm). Fungus infections may also involve the hair and the nails. When the infection is confined to the skin the involvement is superficial and can be treated locally with a cream. When the hair and nails are involved, however, the problem becomes more complex and a combination of oral and topical therapy may be necessary.

### RATIONALE FOR TREATMENT

Fungus infections of the skin are usually treated when they cause itchiness and inflammation or unsightly skin spots, or when they begin to destroy the hair or nails. Although small areas of fungus infection may resolve on their own, your physician will usually elect to treat most fungus infections of the skin because of the potential to cause significant damage to hair or nails and also because of the possibility that the infection can spread to other children.

## HOME TREATMENT

There is no effective home treatment for fungus infections of the skin. The itchy skin lesions may be treated with cold soaks or with calamine lotion. Antifungal medicines, however, are required to kill the fungus and stop the infection.

## TREATMENT AFTER CONSULTING YOUR PHYSICIAN

As has already been mentioned, fungus infection of the skin involves the outer layers and can be effectively treated with topical medicines. The most common antifungal creams in use are miconazole (Micatin), haloprogin (Halotex), clotrimazole (Lotrimin), and tolnaftate (Tinactin, which is available without a prescription). These creams are effective within one to three weeks and have almost no side effects. The choice of cream depends on what kind of fungus is causing the infection. Your doctor can determine this by making an educated guess of what is the most likely fungus to grow in a particular site, or by culturing the fungus in a special fungus culture medium. Occasionally the fungus causing a particular infection will not be covered by the chosen cream, and either a culture will have to be done to determine what the organism is, or another cream must be tried.

Infection of the hair and scalp (tinea capitis) is a fungus infection that involves not only the scalp but also the growing hair. The major difficulty with fungus infections of the hair and scalp is that the fungus becomes incorporated inside the growing hair and becomes inaccessible to topical treatment. When this occurs, it is necessary to give antifungal medicines by mouth so that they can be absorbed into the bloodstream and from there diffuse into the skin and the hair. The most commonly used medicine of this type is griseofulvin. Although griseofulvin is an effective medicine, treatment is long, usually requiring three to four doses a day for up to six weeks to completely eradicate the fungus from the hair. Some physicians will also employ topical antifungal medicines with the griseofulvin to treat any funguses that reside in the superficial layers of the scalp.

Fungus infections of the nails are even more difficult to treat. Here again the fungus becomes incorporated into the nail and is inaccessible to topical treatment. Moreover, because the nail is not rich with blood vessels, it is difficult for the griseofulvin to reach the site of infection. Therapy of the nail should be approached with the realization that even prolonged administration of griseofulvin may not lead to a cure; and even if there is a cure, relapse is not uncommon. Effective therapy can take up to five to six months for fingernails and six to eighteen months for toenails. In fact, toenails respond so poorly to griseofulvin that it is often necessary to remove the nail before the infection can be eliminated.

### IS THE TREATMENT WORKING?

Superficial fungus infections of the skin will usually respond in three to four days to topical treatment. Complete resolution of the skin infection occurs within one to three weeks. If there is no improvement in a skin infection within one week or cure of the infection by one month, it is possible that the infection is caused by a fungus that is not treated by the chosen antifungal cream or that the condition of the skin is caused by some problem other than fungus. As has been mentioned, treatment of the scalp and hair is a more prolonged course with resolution of the infection by six to twelve weeks. Even after the infection has been treated, you may still notice some residual baldness in your child's scalp for several more weeks. If hair does not begin to grow back by this time, you should consult your physician. Infections of the nails take an extremely long time to treat and results may not be noted for anywhere from six to eighteen months.

# Infestations

Two infestations of the skin, lice and scabies, currently afflict children in near epidemic proportions. Effective treatment of these conditions is intimately tied to a knowledge of how these organisms live and die on your child's skin. Unfortunately, there is considerable confusion in this area on the part of parents and physicians alike. We will in this section attempt to shed some light on the natural life cycle of these bugs and how the cycle is affected by the various treatment regimens.

## LICE

### DESCRIPTION

Lice can infest the scalp hair, the skin, and in the older child the pubic hair (pediculosis). Infestation of the skin and the pubic hair, however, is rare in children and we will therefore confine most of our discussion to infestations of the head or head lice. Children contract head lice through close contact in play, through shared clothing or brushes, and to a lesser extent from bedding or towels. In the average case of head lice, no more than ten mature lice are present at one time on the scalp. These lice, however, can live for up to one month on the scalp and can lay up to ten eggs a day. These eggs, sometimes called ova, become firmly attached to the hair. When this occurs, the eggs and their cement-like attachments are called nits and hatch in about seven to nine days. Even if the egg is killed by the appropriate treatment the nit will not fall off the hair. It is fixed to the hair shaft by a strong cement secreted by the louse and either has to be physically removed or will disappear when the hair naturally falls out. What this means for you as a parent is that first because there are so few head lice present with the average infestation you may see only the nits and not the lice when you examine your child's scalp. Second, even after the appropriate treatment kills the lice and the eggs, the nits will persist, until the hairs naturally fall out.

### RATIONALE FOR TREATMENT

There are few things more disturbing to a parent or to a child than bugs in the hair. Although the infestation itself is not serious, it will cause persistent itching and scaling of the scalp and is highly contagious to other adults and children. Moreover, if you wish to be persona non grata at the next PTA meeting, just let it be known that you allowed your child to return to school with untreated head lice.

## HOME TREATMENT

There is no effective home treatment of head lice. In the day and age of modern medicines to treat head lice, the practice of shaving the scalp, pouring gasoline on the scalp, and other home remedies can only be condemned.

## TREATMENT AFTER CONSULTING YOUR PHYSICIAN

The physician will be able to offer you two effective medicines to treat head lice. The most commonly employed medicine is a pesticide called Lindane (gamma benzene hexachloride, Kwell). It comes in a shampoo and should be worked into a lather and left on the scalp for five minutes and then rinsed off. Occasionally, a second treatment twenty-four hours later is recommended for more severe infestations, but this is usually not necessary. Remember, even after the treatment is completed the nits will still remain on the scalp. At this point you may either wait for them to disappear as the hair naturally falls out and is replaced by new hair, or you may wash the hair with one part vinegar and one part water in an attempt to loosen up the nits. Some parents have also recommended soaking a comb in vinegar and removing the nits this way. The other commonly employed medicine is pyrethins (A-200), which is available without a prescription at your local pharmacy. This medication is applied to the scalp for ten minutes and then rinsed off. It should not be used more than twice in twenty-four hours. Care should be taken to avoid contact with the eyes.

Much has been written about the potential toxicity of Lindane to the brain. The toxicity of this medication has been demonstrated in animals exposed to extremely high doses of the medicine and in the rare infant who has had the medication inappropriately applied over a large portion of his or her body, usually over previously inflamed skin. What is important to remember is that no damage to the brain has been demonstrated when this medication has been applied in recommended doses on normal skin. Comparable toxicities to pyrethins have not been reported. This medication, however, can cause corneal ulcers when it comes in contact with the eye. It takes potent medicines to kill head lice. However, if these medicines are used in the recommended way only when the diagnosis is confirmed, we feel that the potential for harm to your child is extremely small. In addition to treatment with medicines, your physician may recommend washing of all combs, brushes, and bedding in very hot water. Your physician may also recommend delousing of clothes. If this is the case, it will be necessary to boil the clothes and steam iron the seams or to take them to the dry cleaner. Because of the highly contagious nature of head lice, your physician may also recommend that all members of the family be treated regardless of the presence or absence of lice or nits.

## SCABIES

### DESCRIPTION

Scabies, like head lice, is a common affliction affecting children today. Unlike head lice, scabies is not an easy diagnosis for your physician to make. It is next to impossible to identify the insect on the skin, and unfortunately this is the only way your physician can positively make the diagnosis. Be tolerant of your physician if the prescribed treatment does not work; this is not because the wrong medicine was prescribed but rather because it was difficult to make the correct diagnosis.

### RATIONALE FOR TREATMENT

Scabies is not a serious infestation of the skin, but it can cause intense itching and discomfort for your child. Moreover, the itching can lead to scratching of the skin and this can lead to impetigo. If this was not enough reason to treat it, scabies is also contagious and can readily be spread to other children and to other members of the family.

## HOME TREATMENT

There is no effective home treatment for scabies.

## TREATMENT AFTER CONSULTING YOUR PHYSICIAN

There are two commonly employed medicines to treat scabies. The most frequently used medicine in older children is gamma benzene hexachloride—Kwell lotion. Treatment of scabies with this medicine requires that you apply the lotion all over the body from the neck down; leave it on for six to eight hours. This single treatment is effective in most cases of scabies, but for some more serious infestations retreatment may be necessary, three to seven days later. Retreatment with Kwell should not be done more than once without further consulting your physician. Because of the potential toxicities of Kwell, many physicians do not recommend using it on children under the age of two years because of the greater tendency for the medicine to be absorbed the younger the child.

Scabies may also be effectively treated with crotamiton cream (Eurax). This preparation should be massaged into the skin of the whole body, working from the chin down. Contact with the eyes, mouth, and the openings of the urethra and anus should be avoided. Two applications should be made at twenty-four hour intervals and a cleansing bath should be taken forty-eight hours following the last application. This treatment will be effective in most cases of scabies, but in a few resistant cases treatment may need to be repeated one week later or an alternative drug used. Again, retreatment should occur only once without further consultation with your physician. Because there has been no reported potential brain toxicity with it, crotamiton is the recommended antiscabies drug for children under the age of two years. Your physician may also recommend treating close friends, family members, pets, and other animals regardless of whether they are symptomatic in order to prevent a relapse and reinfection.

An alternative is to treat your child and then treat other

members of the household only if reinfection or treatment failure occurs. Many physicians will also recommend that linen should be washed in hot water or dry cleaned to prevent reinfection.

### Is the Treatment Working?

You will know that the scabies treatment is working by a decrease in the itching over a three to five day period. In some cases, however, an allergic reaction develops to the mite and the itching may persist for several weeks in spite of treatment. If this occurs, you should consult your physician. New spots or bites should not develop, and there should be a slow disappearance of the bites that are present. It should be remembered that the disappearance of all the bite marks may take several weeks. If the treatment fails, consider the possibility of reinfection from friends, pets, other household members, linen, bedding, or towels. If all these have been accounted for, retreatment may be necessary. If retreatment fails, you should consult your physician again and consider the possibility that an incorrect diagnosis has been made.

---

# Diaper Rashes

### Description

Diaper rashes are among the most common skin conditions affecting infants. The causes of diaper rash are multiple, and at any given time more than one or even all these causes may contribute to the problem. Simply said, a diaper rash is the response of the skin to a changing or abnormal environment in the diaper area. The important elements in this environment are the dampness, heat, and irritant chemicals in the urine and stool or diarrhea fluid. The presence of bacteria or yeast, and possible allergic reactions to rubber and plastic, diaper detergents, and disinfectants may also play a role. Occasionally the diaper rash may be part of a more widespread skin disease affecting your child such as seborrheic dermatitis or impetigo. In most cases, however, the rash is the result of this complex interaction of elements in the diaper environment.

### RATIONALE FOR TREATMENT

Most diaper rashes will disappear when abnormal changes in the diaper environment return to normal. An example of this is diarrhea. Diarrhea will commonly cause a red irritation of your baby's bottom that is refractory to most conventional treatments until the diarrhea disappears. Occasionally a diaper rash does not respond to simple measures like waiting for a change in the bowel habits or more frequent changes of the diaper. Instead it becomes progressively irritated and red, causing discomfort for your infant. When this occurs, more intensive treatment is required both in changing the diaper environment and in eliminating possible offending agents such as bacteria or yeast.

### HOME TREATMENT

Because of the many factors involved in a diaper rash, there is no single treatment that yields a quick and effective response. The general approach to treatment involves first altering the environment to remove possible irritating conditions, and if this is not sufficient then to turn to your physician for medicines aimed directly at reducing inflammation or killing such organisms as yeast and bacteria. Altering the diaper environment can include keeping the area as free of urine and stool as possible through frequent diaper changes, avoiding the use of occlusive rubber pants that increase the temperature and humidity of the diaper area, and exposing the diaper area as much as possible to the open air. The application of a bland protective ointment or cream such as Desitin or Diaparene will prevent possible irritants in the urine or stool from reaching the skin. Some physicians and parents recommend rinsing cloth diapers in a dilute acid (one ounce of vinegar to one gallon of water) to reduce the irritating alkalinity imparted by soap and detergent residues. If these efforts are unsuccessful over a five to seven day period, or if the rash is getting worse, it may be that yeast is involved or that the degree of inflammation is so severe that it cannot respond to simple changes in the environment. In this situation, consultation with your physician is necessary.

### TREATMENT AFTER CONSULTING YOUR PHYSICIAN

The most common reason for a refractory diaper rash is overgrowth of yeast in the diaper area. This usually produces a characteristic rash that your physician can readily recognize. If this is the case, your physician will recommend the application of an antiyeast cream. The most commonly employed creams are nystatin (Mycostatin), clotrimazole (Lotrimin), or miconazole (Micatin). Nystatin has the advantage of being less expensive and equally effective. Moreover, it comes in a powder form that can often be more easily applied when the skin is swollen and weeping. If the degree of inflammation is significant, your physician will frequently suggest a mild steroid cream such as 1% hydrocortisone. If this is used as directed, side effects from the treatment are minimal. Steroids do not eliminate the cause of the rash and on occasion may worsen the rash if given without a needed antimicrobial cream. You should avoid the temptation to treat diaper rashes with steroid medication without first consulting your physician. Almost all diaper rashes will get better without steroids, but a severe diaper rash usually will get better faster with them.

### IS THE TREATMENT WORKING?

With the appropriate treatment regimen you should notice improvement in the diaper rash in a period of five to seven days. Complete disappearance of all signs of a severe diaper rash may, however, take several weeks. If the diaper rash does not respond in this period of time you should consult your physician, for the rash may be a manifestation of a more complex skin condition.

# Allergic Reactions

Your child's skin is sensitive to allergic reactions. His or her skin may come in direct contact with a substance that produces an allergic reaction such as poison oak or ivy, or the skin may be the target of an allergic reaction to something that has been inhaled or swallowed, such as penicillin. In this section we discuss both types of allergic reactions and let you know when to treat, and what treatments are available to you at home and in the doctor's office.

## CONTACT DERMATITIS

### DESCRIPTION

Contact dermatitis is just that; it is an inflammation of the skin caused by contact with a substance that either directly irritates the skin or induces an allergic reaction. The irritating kind of contact dermatitis is usually caused by repeated or prolonged exposure to soaps, detergents, and solvents. Allergic contact dermatitis, on the other hand, involves an allergic reaction of the skin that can take place after only one exposure. There is usually a period of five to twenty-one days between the exposure and the development of the rash. This makes the identification of the offending agent very difficult if not impossible. Irritant and allergic contact dermatitis are unfortunately indistinguishable in their appearance. Treatment of both conditions, however, is essentially the same. Thus, when we talk about the treatment of allergic contact dermatitis this will also include the treatment of irritant contact dermatitis. When certain areas such as the hands are involved, irritant contact dermatitis should be considered, and irritants should be searched for in the environment.

### RATIONALE FOR TREATMENT

Treatment of contact dermatitis depends upon the amount of misery caused by the allergic reaction. In some cases, brief exposure to an allergic substance may cause only a mild itchy rash that will disappear in three to five days. On the other hand, intense or repeated exposure to an allergic substance may cause considerable inflammation, swelling, oozing, and itchiness of the skin. In both situations, provided that there is no repeated exposure to the allergic substance, the condition will resolve without serious complications. How you treat your child will depend on how miserable he or she is and how long you can put up with that misery. Some children are able to tolerate a severe allergic reaction to poison oak without any treatment; for others, the slightest itchy allergic rash will drive them to distraction. It is the compassionate parent who bases the decision to treat not on the appearance of the skin, but rather on the degree of discomfort experienced by the child.

## HOME TREATMENT

Much can be done to treat contact dermatitis at home without having to travel to the doctor's office. In those situations when the skin is red, itchy, oozing, and swollen, much of the discomfort can be minimized by soaking the skin with wet dressings. A convenient solution for a wet dressing is Burow's solution (aluminum acetate). This is available over the counter in convenient powder packets or tablets or Domeboro powder or tablets. One packet is dissolved in a pint of water and soft gauze, linen, or old handkerchiefs or shirts are dipped in the solution, wrung out, and wrapped around the affected area six to eight times. Optimally the dressings should be changed every ten to fifteen minutes for thirty minutes to two hours. This should be repeated three times a day. This treatment helps to dry the skin and greatly reduce the oozing and blistering. This also makes it easier to apply topical medicine should it be needed. For widespread involvement soaking can be done in the bathtub. A commonly used bath preparation is the oatmeal bath. This can be purchased over the counter as Aveeno Oatmeal Bath or Aveeno with Oil Oatmeal Bath. One cup of Aveeno is mixed with two cups of cold tapwater and added to a tub half-full of tepid water. The duration of the bath should not exceed thirty minutes. Starch baths can also be used by mixing two cups of hydrolyzed starch with four cups of cold tapwater and adding the paste to a half-full tub of warm water. The application of calamine lotion has been frequently used by parents to reduce the itching of allergic reactions. (Do not use Caladryl, which may irritate the skin.) This lotion works by cooling and drying the skin and minimizing the itching. Aspirin and antihistamines sold over the counter may also help in alleviating the discomfort of contact dermatitis.

### TREATMENT AFTER CONSULTING YOUR PHYSICIAN

When the previously described home treatments are not sufficient to alleviate your child's misery, your physician will frequently turn to the use of steroids to reduce the inflammation, and ultimately the itching and pain. For mild cases of inflammation, the best way to administer these steroids is topically in a cream, ointment, or lotion. There are a number of preparations of topical steroids varying in strength, consistency (cream, ointment, and lotion), and cost. In general, your physician will start with a more potent (and more expensive) steroid cream to immediately reduce the inflammation, and then maintain the inflammation at a low level with a less potent steroid. The more potent steroid preparations are available only by prescription. The steroid available over the counter in your pharmacy (0.5% hydrocortisone) is, except for very mild cases, not potent enough to relieve the inflammation quickly. After your physician has prescribed a topical steroid for your child, you should apply it in a thin layer (this is one situation where more is not better, only more expensive) two or three times a day.

Treatment with topical steroids is a quick and effective means of reducing the inflammation in allergic contact dermatitis. These preparations, however, are not without side effects. Prolonged administration of topical steroids over large areas of the skin can lead to increased absorption of the steroids from the skin to the rest of the body. This bodywide absorption can lead to serious side effects including the suppression or turning off of important hormones in the body, which after treatment may turn on slowly, leaving the body vulnerable to illness. Prolonged use of topical steroids can also produce serious side effects in the skin. These include changes in the small blood vessels or capillaries of the skin, purple marks or stria in the skin, and atrophy or fading away of the skin. In order to minimize these side effects, you should work with your physician to reduce the potency and duration of treatment with topical steroids as quickly as is possible without causing undue discomfort for your child. Although the duration of topical steroid treatment should be as short as possible, be careful not to stop the treatment too abruptly, for this may lead to a flaring of the reaction all over again. To avoid this phenomenon, many physicians recommend tapering the steroid medicine slowly by decreasing both the frequency of application and the potency of the preparation.

Reducing the itchiness of the dermatitis can also be aided by the use of antihistamines. It is unclear to us whether the major effects of these medicines is due to the blocking of the chemical histamine in the skin that may be responsible for the itching, or if the antihistamine just makes the child so sleepy that he or she does not care about the itching. Regardless of the mechanism, these medicines can be useful particularly at bedtime, when itching and scratching are most severe. This is one situation when an antihistamine with a strong sedative or drowsiness effect is the best choice. A commonly used example of this type of antihistamine is diphenhydramine hydrochloride (Benadryl). Occasionally the prescribed dose of antihistamine will not be sufficent to diminish your child's itching. In this case, it is important to work with your physician to adjust your child's dose to achieve the desired results without undue side effects.

For those cases of severe allergic contact dermatitis when more areas of the skin are affected and the swelling and blistering more marked, your child may be disabled to the point where he or she is unable to go to school. In this case, the use of potent steroids given by mouth or by injection may be warranted. This route of administration allows the blood stream to deliver the steroid to the site of inflammation quickly and effectively. These steroids are usually given in high doses for three to seven days and then tapered off to reduce the possibility of the side effects previously discussed. Again, there is the risk of the inflammation flaring if the steroids are tapered too rapidly.

## Is the Treatment Working?

You will know that the treatment regimen is working when you observe a reduction in the itchiness and redness of the skin within twenty-four hours. New areas of dermatitis may appear after the therapy has been started. This is because the timing of the appearance of the dermatitis is related to the amount of exposure to the causative substance. Those areas that were exposed to large amounts of the offending substance will be the first to become inflamed whereas those areas that were less exposed may become inflamed up to five days later. Because of this, it may appear that the dermatitis is spreading, but in reality the skin is reacting to different degrees of exposure. Moderate to severe contact dermatitis can take three weeks or longer to resolve. It is imperative that you closely follow your physician's instruction with regard to steroid therapy during this period to ensure that the inflammation does not flare and that no serious side effects ensue.

In cases of repeated allergic contact dermatitis, efforts should be made to identify and avoid the offending substance. This, however, can be a difficult task and if the offending substance remains unknown, referral to a physician familiar with patch testing may be useful. In patch testing, potential allergic substances are applied to your child's skin on an adhesive bandage and the skin is examined for an allergic reaction. If an allergic reaction appears, this may identify a possible causative agent. Once the offending substance has been identified, some physicians recommend a hypersensitization or the adminstration of the offending substances in small amounts over a period of time with the hope of building up resistance to inflammation. This treatment has been most widely used for poison oak and ivy. We feel that the benefits of this treatment are usually negligible and not worth the effort of the painful and prolonged series of injections.

## ALLERGIC REACTIONS OF THE SKIN OTHER THAN CONTACT DERMATITIS

Allergic reactions of the skin other than contact dermatitis take two forms. The first is a late-appearing allergic reaction characterized by a red rash all over the body occurring five to seven days after starting a new medicine or ingesting a new food. The second type of allergic reaction is characterized by the immediate development of a red rash over most parts of the body in response to taking a medicine or ingesting a particular food substance, or in response to a change in the environment, such as cold and heat. This type of reaction is frequently referred to as hives or urticaria. This latter condition may be chronic, or may be part of a more serious allergic reaction.

### LATE-APPEARING ALLERGIC REACTION

**DESCRIPTION**

The rash associated with this type of allergic reaction usually appears within one week after exposure to the causative agent. The rash may appear after the first exposure, or it may inexplicably occur after many exposures. This type of reaction will usually disappear within two to three weeks, whether or not the offending food or drug has been stopped.

**RATIONALE FOR TREATMENT**

The most obvious treatment for this type of allergic reaction is the elimination of the offending substance. If, however, your child is taking a medicine for a specific illness, it may be more important for him or her to finish the treatment than it is to eliminate the medicine. This latter decision may cause the rash to persist for a few days longer, but it is important to remember that the rash would still persist for up to two to three weeks regardless of whether the medicine is stopped or not. You should consult with your physician about what to do if a rash of this type occurs.

### HOME TREATMENT

The hallmark of this type of rash is itchiness. Treatment of the symptom can be the same as was described for contact dermatitis, with the exception that topical steroids are rarely used.

### TREATMENT AFTER CONSULTING YOUR PHYSICIAN

Occasionally an allergic reaction may be particularly severe, causing considerable discomfort for your child. When this occurs, your physician may recommend the use of systemic steroids for a short period of time to reduce the troublesome symptoms and to allow your child to resume normal activities.

### IS THE TREATMENT WORKING?

It is important to remember that even when you have removed the offending substance the rash may still persist for two to three weeks. Treatment with local preparations, such as calamine lotion or oatmeal baths, may reduce the symptoms caused by the rash, but it will not ultimately affect the course of the allergic reaction. This is also true for the use of systemic steroids. Although the steroids will cause a decrease in the amount of symptoms experienced by your child, the allergic reaction must still run its course before it can completely resolve. If you should stop the steroids before the course has resolved, there is a good chance that the allergic reaction would flare again.

## HIVES OR URTICARIA

### DESCRIPTION

Hives or urticaria can occur in response to drugs, food, or food additives. Urticaria can also occur for nonallergic reasons such as infection, colds, temperature changes, exercise, emotions, trauma, or pressure to the skin. Because of the many causes of urticaria, the offending agent or process usually cannot be determined in up to 80–90% of cases.

### RATIONALE FOR TREATMENT

Treatment for hives is warranted when the cause can be identified and removed, or when the associated itching is so intense that it is causing your child considerable discomfort.

### TREATMENT AT HOME

The itching of urticaria can be diminished by using the topical measures that were described above for contact dermatitis. Oatmeal baths, calamine lotions, and wet dressings of cool water without the aluminum acetate can go a long way in relieving the symptoms. Aspirin and antihistamines purchased over the counter can also be helpful.

### TREATMENT AFTER CONSULTING YOUR PHYSICIAN

If the previously described measures are not effective, your physician can prescribe antihistamines to help reduce the symptoms. If the urticaria is part of a more severe allergic reaction, shots of epinephrine and systemic steroids may be necessary and can be life saving.

---

# Acne

### DESCRIPTION

Acne is undoubtedly the easiest skin condition to recognize; nearly everyone has had a personal experience with this problem. Although acne is occasionally seen in infants up to six months of age, it is almost a universal problem of adolescence.

What is a pimple and how is it formed? All pimples begin below the surface of the skin in structures known as sebaceous glands. All of us have millions of these glands, which consist of tiny hairs as well as an area devoted to the production of an oily substance known as sebum. Nobody is quite sure what the function of sebum is; although it plays a role in the courting behavior of some animals, it seems to cause only aggravation for today's teenagers. Ordinarily sebum flows freely to the skin's surface. However, if the outlet of the gland is blocked, as happens when shed cells plug the opening, sebum can build up and in combination with normal bacteria that live in the sebaceous gland produce a reaction resulting in acne.

A variety of skin lesions are seen in the patient with acne. Blackheads, also known as open comedones, consist of tiny cylindrical collections of sebum that have been darkened to a brownish or blackish color by a pigment known as melanin, which comes from the surrounding skin. Blackheads seldom cause problems and often can be removed easily with comedo extractors. Once the opening of the sebaceous gland is blocked, a closed comedo is established. In its mildest form a closed comedo is commonly known as a whitehead. If the opening of the whitehead continues to be blocked a more severe reaction within the skin can occur and lead to the formation of a papule. Closed comedones are often known as time bombs because of the series of chemical reactions that can cause rupture of the walls of the sebaceous gland, leading to the more severe reactions characterized by angry red pustules and ever larger and deeper cyst formation deep within the skin.

Although it is most problematic during the teenage years, acne can begin as early as the age of seven years, and may often persist into the thirties and forties.

## RATIONALE FOR TREATMENT

Acne cannot be treated in the way that an antibiotic can eliminate an infection. However, there are a number of things that can be done to help manage this extremely distressing problem. The first thing to bear in mind when helping your child manage acne is that myths outnumber therapies by at least a factor of ten to one. It is still not uncommon to run into teenagers who believe that certain sexual thoughts or activities may cause or aggravate their skin problem. Similarly there are widespread misconceptions about the role of food in causing acne. Most studies conducted in recent years have *not* been able to show that eating chocolate or nuts or drinking cola is responsible for acne. There are undoubtedly individuals who will experience aggravation of acne with eating a particular type of food. If your son or daughter notices this, by all means encourage him or her to stop eating this food. However, there is no scientific basis for the automatic removal of chocolate, nuts, or other food. Finally, there is the misperception that acne results from a lack of cleanliness and therefore frequent face-washing with the strongest possible soap is a good way to manage acne. Unfortunately, this is not the case. In fact, a number of extremely harsh soaps may be counterproductive; they can cause excessive irritation when used in combination with several of the effective remedies. However, because part of effective treatment is to ensure that sebaceous glands plug up as seldom as possible, mild abrasion of the superficial layers of the skin is a principle underlying acne management. Therefore, use of a wash cloth accompanied by a mild soap, such as Dove or Neutrogena, is recommended. Other forms of treatment are geared at (1) reducing the number of bacteria that reside deep within the skin, and (2) altering some of the chemical reactions that occur within the sebaceous gland.

## HOME TREATMENT

In addition to dispelling some of the myths about acne, there are many other things that can be accomplished at home. Acne may be fueled by a variety of stresses including tension, lack of sleep, and the pre-menstrual period. Although it is impossible to remove the anxiety that accompanies that big exam, it is important to counter this type of stress with both emotional support and recommendations for a sound night's sleep.

As mentioned previously, diet is seldom the culprit; washing with mild soaps and a wash cloth are suggested and may be sufficient for the child who is fortunate enough to be bothered only by an occasional blackhead.

For most adolescents, over-the-counter therapy will be necessary for good acne control. Fortunately, a number of excellent agents are now available that are quite effective in controlling acne.

Benzoyl peroxide and tretinoin are the most effective preparations currently available and are far better than preparations that contain salicylic acid, sulfur, and resorcinol.

Benzoyl peroxide has been around for nearly sixty years, but only recently has it been formulated in products that have been shown to be quite effective. It acts by causing a mild peeling of the skin and assists in preventing plugging of the sebaceous glands. It also has some activity against bacteria and is able to interfere somewhat with some of the chemical processes involved in the formation of papules and pustules. It can be irritating, especially if used with abrasive soaps, which is why we do not recommend coarse and gritty soaps. As many as 2% of children may be allergic to this product, so it is not for everyone. It also takes a number of weeks before any results will be seen. This is important to bear in mind, for the first few weeks can be discouraging. The goal is to produce a mild dryness of the skin. The best way to achieve this is to begin applications every other day. Begin with the 5% lotion. If there is no skin irritation and the acne persists, it is then possible to increase the concentration to the 10% lotions and go to an every-day basis. The most potent forms are available in gels.

Some cosmetics can aggravate acne; it is best to avoid them as much as possible, especially when attempting to treat the skin with the agents we have just been discussing. There has been some recent publicity about zinc treatment of acne; this has not yet been proved effective and we do not recommend it. Most diets have sufficient zinc for adequate skin nourishment. Your adolescent's acne will not respond readily to topical treatment if the pimples are large and cystic in nature. Moreover, it is these types of pimples that most often cause scarring. If this situation occurs, you should consult your physician about some of the effective treatments described in the next section.

Acne appears to get better in the summer. Although this is most likely due to increased exposure to sunlight, other factors may be involved. We do not recommend the routine use of sunlamps, the primary effect of which is to induce peeling of the skin, which can be done much more safely by peeling agents such as benzoyl peroxide and tretinoin. Sunlamps can produce severe burns.

### TREATMENT AFTER CONSULTING YOUR PHYSICIAN

If acne continues to be a problem despite adequate home treatment and over-the-counter preparations, your physician will almost certainly prescribe tretinoin or an oral antibiotic.

Tretinoin is also known as retinoic acid and is a form of vitamin A. Tretinoin is also effective but is somewhat more irritating than benzoyl peroxide. We usually begin with benzoyl peroxide, increase its concentration, and then add tretinoin. When used in combination, benzoyl peroxide should be applied during the day and tretinoin at night. The sun will often cause an irritating reaction after tretinoin has been applied. Tretinoin is available in two concentrations of cream (0.05% and 0.1%) as well as a gel and as swabs of liquids. We generally begin with the cream and then advance to the more potent gel and swab forms.

Oral antibiotics have been proved effective and reasonably safe in the management of acne. The most commonly used antibiotic is tetracycline. Often begun in dosages of 500 to 1000 mg daily, tetracycline with success can be reduced to a dosage in the neighborhood of 250 mg every other day. As with most other acne therapies, it works by the prevention of new lesions and will therefore take several weeks before any effect can be seen. Tetracycline causes staining of the teeth in younger children, and should not be used at all on children under the age of eight years; it should be used cautiously on those between the ages of eight and twelve years. It is a safe medication over the age of twelve years, although it frequently causes upset stomach and can be responsible for producing vaginal yeast infections. Erythromycin is an alternative to tetracycline that is also effective, safe, and inexpensive. It also can produce some minor abdominal discomfort. Other antibiotics that are less frequently used, and that should certainly never be the initial drug treatment, include clindamycin and minocycline. The expense and higher frequency of side effects of these antibiotics make them suitable only for cases that have failed to respond to all the therapy previously discussed.

In addition to oral antibiotics, topical antibiotics have also found recent favor in the medical profession. Some preparations, such as topical erythromycin, appear to be effective but have a very short shelf life. Others such as topical clindamycin appear to be no better than less expensive agents such as benzoyl peroxide.

### Is the Treatment Working?

It is unusual not to see improvement of acne after the management approaches that we have discussed. Remember, treatment may not be noticeable for a full month, so don't get discouraged easily. Whether your adolescent is satisfied with the result is another issue. Achieving the perfect unblemished skin of the magazine model is an unachievable goal. Ads portray models as having no pores! The photographer's airbrush has thus created a creature that does not walk the earth.

If any of the previously mentioned treatments create reddening of the skin or excessive peeling it is possible that your child is experiencing an allergic reaction, too high a concentration, or too frequent an application of the medication. Always discuss these situations with your physician. Your physician may decrease the concentration or diminish the timing and frequency of application. If all medication treatment has failed, several office-based procedures are possible—including injection of steroids into large cysts. This is effective though necessary only for severe cases. Although the estrogen content in birth control pills will result in a decrease in sebum production and improvement of acne in some patients, we do not consider the treatment of acne an indication for prescribing birth control pills in women. However, if young women are using birth control pills as their means of contraception, they may notice an improvement in their acne.

# Seborrhea

### DESCRIPTION

Seborrhea is a condition that is normally found in infants (cradle cap) and adolescents (dandruff). In the infant cradle cap consists of yellow oily scales on the scalp and may be associated with a red rash. In the adolescent, dandruff, a flaking of the scalp, is the most common manifestation of seborrhea. Occasionally seborrhea is associated with inflammation (redness, swelling, and oozing of the skin). Then it is called seborrhea dermatitis. Although seborrhea can occur at any point during childhood, it is most common during infancy and adolescence. Increased hormone production during this period leads to the production of an oily substance called sebum, which gives the skin near the scalp its oily appearance. No one is sure why there is increased growth and shedding of cells of the scalp, but it is this shedding that causes the flakes and scales of seborrhea.

### RATIONALE FOR TREATMENT

*Infant* Seborrhea in the infant is most likely a normal developmental phenomenon. It reaches its peak around the third or fourth month of life, and subsides over the next three or four months. What is most commonly seen are yellow greasy-appearing scales on the scalp, eyebrows, and occasionally on the upper chest, underarms, and diaper area. This process may be associated with inflammation of the skin, characterized by redness and a rash. When your infant has seborrhea without inflammation, no treatment is necessary. This normal developmental condition will almost always improve in a period of months. Treatment with various shampoos and lotions may actually irritate your infant's skin, or cause an allergic reaction creating a greater problem than the seborrhea. If there is a bad rash and inflammation of the skin associated with the seborrhea, treatment with steroid creams may be necessary to make your infant more comfortable.

*Adolescent* During adolescence, seborrhea is characterized by scaling and flaking of the scalp. Inflammation of the skin and a rash are much less common. There are two major reasons that lead parents and their adolescent to seek treatment for seborrhea. First, most adolescents are quite concerned about their physical appearance. Even the smallest amount of flaking on the shoulders, or visible in the scalp, may be deemed intolerable. Second, unlike the infant, seborrhea in the adolescent does not routinely disappear and frequently goes on into adulthood. If a decision is made to treat seborrhea, it is important to realize that the various treatments do not eliminate the underlying causes of seborrhea, but eliminate only the flaking on a temporary basis. If the treatment is stopped, the flaking will frequently reappear.

## HOME TREATMENT

*Infant* If your relatives are driving you to distraction about those "ugly yellow crusts" on your infant's scalp and you have to *do something*—we recommend using baby oil on the skin and a soft-bristled tooth brush to remove the scales. This treatment will not "cure" the seborrhea, but it will improve its appearance.

*Adolescent* When the decision has been made to treat your adolescent's seborrhea, there are several shampoos available designed to slow the growth rate of the scalp skin cells and diminish the shedding and flaking. The shampoos that are most effective contain the active ingredient selenium sulfide (Selsun Blue) or zinc pyrithione (Head and Shoulders, Danex, Zincon). Less effective are shampoos containing salicylic acid-sulfur combination (Ionil, Meted, Sebulex, and Vanseb). The least effective are tar shampoos (DHS-T, Ionil-T, Pentrax, Sebutone, and Zetar), which do not decrease the rate of shedding. These preparations are available over the counter in most pharmacies. Be sure to closely follow the directions, for improper use can lead to irritation of the scalp.

### TREATMENT AFTER CONSULTING YOUR PHYSICIAN

When significant inflammation occurs, or when an extensive rash is present, treatment with more potent concentrations of selenium sulfide or treatment with topical corticosteroids may be necessary. In most cases 1% hydrocortisone cream will suffice for the infant. In the adolescent it may be necessary to use a topical steroid lotion or spray to control inflammation.

### IS THE TREATMENT WORKING?

In the infant, most seborrhea will improve with time no matter what you do. Scrubbing of the scalp with mineral oil will remove the scales quickly, but it is not unusual for them to return in a period of days or weeks. Treatment of inflamed seborrhea with topical steroids should produce a reduction in redness in one to two days, and an improvement in the rash in one to two weeks. For the adolescent, proper therapy with the appropriate shampoos should produce some improvement in two to three applications. The degree of response will vary from adolescent to adolescent, with complete eradication of seborrhea being the exception rather than the rule.

# Eczema (Atopic Dermatitis)

### DESCRIPTION

Atopic dermatitis is perhaps the most common chronic skin condition affecting infants and children. Although allergic symptoms such as a runny nose and wheezing are strongly associated with atopic dermatitis, there is no good evidence to indicate that it is "allergic" in character. Children with atopic dermatitis have skin which responds to changes in the environment, allergic substances in foods, and emotional stress, with intense itching. Atopic skin also has increased tendency to swell and ooze when scratched. A vicious cycle is thus established in which changes in the environment lead to intense itching of the skin and scratching leads to swelling, oozing, and inflammation and eventually to more itching. Atopic dermatitis is a condition that may be chronic and recurring; any therapy directed at atopic dermatitis can be expected to alleviate the symptoms but will not cure the basic abnormality of the skin.

Atopic dermatitis is a condition that presents itself in different ways at different ages. During infancy (two months to two years) the dermatitis is characterized by inflammation of the skin with pimples, blisters, and occasionally swelling and oozing. The pattern of distribution during this age is also quite characteristic, with the dermatitis occurring primarily on the cheeks, neck, shoulders, and occasionally the diaper area. During childhood (four to ten years), the disease is characterized by less inflammation and increased buildup of the layers of the skin to give it a leathery appearance. Here the areas primarily affected are the insides of the arms at the elbow joint, and behind the knees.

In adolescents there is a buildup of the skin to give a dry, leathery appearance and a minimal amount of inflammation. Here the areas primarily affected are the hands and feet, although the insides of the arms and the backs of the knees may also be involved.

## RATIONALE FOR TREATMENT

Atopic determatitis requires treatment when itching and scratching produce inflammation, swelling, and infection of the skin. Treatment is also required when continuous scratching leads to a buildup of skin (lichenification) that causes an unsightly, leathery appearance. If the atopic dermatitis is only causing a mild rash behind your infant's neck or a minimal amount of itching on your child's arms and legs, treatment is not necessary. The decision to treat should be made according to how miserable your child is, and how much damage is being done to the skin.

### HOME TREATMENT

When inflammation is a prominent characteristic of your child's atopic dermatitis—the skin is red, swollen, oozing, and itchy—a wet dressing of Burow's solution (see the section in this chapter on Contact Dermatitis) and total body oatmeal baths can be applied. In those cases when inflammation is minimal and the prominent characteristics are dry, itchy, or thickened skin, symptoms can be minimized by (1) keeping the environment at a low normal temperature and high humidity to prevent evaporation of water from the skin, and (2) not bathing excessively with drying detergent soaps. Use of a cleansing agent such as cetaphil or a nondetergent soap such as Dove will prevent the leeching of oils from the skin and keep the skin from drying out. Frequent use of lubricating lotions and creams should be encouaged to help retain moisture in the skin. These preparations are best applied when the skin is moist. A good lubricating lotion can be inexpensively made by combining Crisco and glycerine. If this is not palatable to you, such commercial preparations as Keri, Lubriderm (lotions), Keri, Nivea (creams), and Eucerin (creamy paste) are available at your pharmacy.

### TREATMENT AFTER CONSULTING YOUR PHYSICIAN

When the inflammation accompanying atopic dermatitis is particularly severe, the use of topical steroids may be necessary. Steroid treatment is usually started with one of the more potent topical steroids, which for severe cases may be applied as frequently as six times a day. This will usually suppress the inflammation quickly, stop the itching, and break the vicious cycle. Once this has been accomplished, your physician should then switch to a less potent steroid for more long-term treatment of the inflammation. Antihistamines can be given by mouth to suppress the itchiness; they will also make it easier to sleep at night. In very severe cases of atopic dermatitis, steroids need to be given systematically. Occasionally hospitalization is necessary for intensive therapy.

In those cases of atopic dermatitis when inflammation is minimal and the condition is characterized by dry, itchy, thickened skin, a low-potency steroid preparation (usually an ointment to help hold in the moisture) will be prescribed to help reduce any residual inflammation and alleviate the itching. Many physicians feel that the skin in atopic dermatitis is a fertile growing ground for bacteria, and that in most cases of atopic dermatitis there is an overgrowth of bacteria that worsens the condition. When this occurs, an antibiotic, usually erythromycin (this drug is chosen because of its ability to effectively reach the skin) is prescribed. Although this treatment has not been well proved scientifically, we feel that for cases of atopic dermatitis when there is moderate to severe inflammation a trial of antibiotics can be a useful adjunct to overall therapy. Sometimes acute infections will develop which require oral antibiotic therapy.

The role of allergy in atopic dermatitis is controversial. Most physicians and allergists feel that particular foods play an important role in precipitating atopic dermatitis in infants and toddlers. Because of this, food elimination diets (this is a diet where all the potentially allergy-producing foodstuffs are eliminated and then added back in one by one) are often prescribed first to identify the offending food and then to eliminate it. Many dermatologists, however, are not as enthusiastic as other physicians about the usefulness of a good elimination diet. They prescribe it only after all other therapies have failed. Undoubtedly, the truth lies somewhere in between these two viewpoints. We feel that a food elimination diet is not harmful to infants; it may produce dramatic results. Because the diet is relatively easy to comply with in infants and toddlers, we feel that it is worth a try in cases of moderate to severe dermatitis. There is, on the other hand, no proof that allergic substances in the environment other than ingested foods play an important role in atopic dermatitis. We feel that there is no role for allergy skin tests or allergy shots in the treatment of atopic dermatitis.

### IS THE TREATMENT WORKING?

In atopic dermatitis, knowing when the treatment is working can be a difficult problem. This can be a chronic, recurring disease, and its precipitants and exacerbants are poorly defined. It is possible that your child will get worse in spite of appropriate therapy or better regardless of the therapy. Because of this, it is important that you do not feel directly responsible (or feel that your child is directly responsible) for any relapses or worsening of symptoms. This is still a poorly understood condition that often runs a course of its own despite our best advised remedies. Keeping these considerations in mind, it is reasonable to expect some improvement in your child's skin within a five to seven day period. The inflammatory components of this condition should resolve within this given time period, but the lichenification or the thickening of the skin may take several weeks or months to disappear. Response to the food elimination diet may take up to three to four weeks. Addition of an offending foodstuff into the diet should precipitate symptoms again within one to three days.

Again, keep in mind that relapses are the rule. Expect them, don't be discouraged by them, and be ready to treat them when they occur. Frequently your child's atopic dermatitis will shift between acute inflammatory condition and a chronic dry, thickened condition. This necessitates constant tuning of your therapy and adjustment to the given conditions. Here close commuication with your physician can be most helpful.

# Sunburn

### DESCRIPTION

With our current passion for outdoor life, and tanned

healthy-looking skin, it is not unusual that some children and adolescents will overexpose themselves to sunlight and sunlamps and become sunburned. Sunburn is the result of excessive exposure to ultraviolet light from the sun or sunlamps. This light is not screened out by thin clouds on an overcast day; and hats and umbrellas do not provide adequate protection because much of this exposure is from sunlight reflected off water, sidewalks, or snow. Blue-eyed persons, redheads, blondes, and frecklers withstand sun exposure poorly. A fair-skinned person spending fifteen to twenty minutes in the noonday sun at the latitude of Philadelphia or Denver will receive a mild sunburn. A sunburn can range from a mild redness appearing two to four hours after exposure, to vivid redness, with swelling and blistering of the skin, chills, nausea, and fever. Extreme exposure to the sun is more than just a tourist's hazard; it can result in a serious burn.

## RATIONALE FOR TREATMENT

The best treatment for sunburn is prevention. Although tanned skin may appear healthy, there is nothing healthy about prolonged exposure of your skin to the sun. Not only may it result in a burn, it will also leech important oils from your skin, leading to drying and wrinkling. It is also a risk factor for the development of skin cancer. Once sunburn has occurred, treatment may be necessary to reduce the discomfort and to minimize the damaging effects of the burn on the skin.

## HOME TREATMENT

*Prevention*   Sun protection medicines are available over the counter in most drug stores that are as useful and effective as any sunscreen available. The most commonly available sun lotions and sunscreens contain para-aminobenzoic acid (PABA) as their active ingredient. The most effective preparations contain 5% PABA, with lesser concentrations screening out lesser amounts of ultraviolet light. A second group of sunscreens contain as their active ingredient benzopherone. Although these products protect against a wider spectrum of light, they are less effective than PABA in the important part of the ultraviolet light spectrum. They wash off easily and need to be frequently applied. The third group of products called sunshades contain opaque substances such as zinc oxide. Although these are the most effective sun protection agents, they are messy and cosmetically undesirable.

Sunscreens are evaluated by a number known as the Sun Protective Factor (SPF). This factor is a measure of the amount of energy necessary to produce a mild burn on the skin. It has been recommended that sunscreen products be labeled with an SPF number. Five categories have been proposed: SPF 2–4, minimal protection from sunburn but permit suntanning; SPF 4–6, moderate protection, but permit suntanning; SPF 6–8, extra protection from sunburn and permit limited suntanning; SPF 8–15, maximum protection sunburn and permit suntanning; over 15, most protection from sunburn and permit no suntanning. It should be noted that these are laboratory determinations which frequently overestimate the degree of protection.

If a sunburn does occur, cool tap-water compresses applied for twenty minutes and aspirin or acetaminophen are about as effective as any treatment. The only active ingredient that is as effective in over-the-counter sunburn preparations is 20% benzocaine (Americaine). This can be tried if the previously described remedies do not work. The danger with using them is that they may cause an allergic skin reaction on your child. If you suspect that a serious burn may have taken place (e.g., your adolescent fell asleep under the sunlamp) contact your physician right away. This is one situation where early treatment can make a difference.

#### TREATMENT AFTER CONSULTING YOUR PHYSICIAN

For moderate to severe burns your physician may elect to treat with topical corticosteroid lotion or cream. Severe burns may require large doses of steroids by mouth, as well as cool compresses and stronger medications for pain. Remember, a serious sunburn is not something that is easily treated at home; your physician should be consulted.

### Is the Treatment Working?

The ideal sunscreen should allow you to tan without burning. This unfortunately involves a careful balance of the strength of sunscreen, and amount and intensity of exposure. In other words, what worked for one trip to the beach may not work for the next trip.

Treatment for sunburn is effective when it hurts less. For more serious burns treatment should bring about reduction in redness and pain within twenty-four hours.

# CHAPTER TWENTY-SEVEN

# Asthma

## DESCRIPTION

ASTHMA IS A VERY common problem; as many as 5 percent of children may be troubled with recurrent episodes. Children with asthma have a respiratory system with air passages that are unusually sensitive to certain irritants. Their airways respond to these irritants by narrowing that is caused by three simultaneous events: (1) airway muscles constricting, (2) swelling of airway linings, and (3) the appearance of mucus, which clogs the airways. A narrow airway means that a child must work harder to breathe, especially to exhale (breathe out). Symptoms include difficulty breathing, wheezing, coughing, becoming short of breath while exercising, and a tight feeling in the chest.

Many of us respond to irritants, such as chemical fumes, with airway narrowing. However, children with asthma have a more exaggerated response to common irritants and respond to certain items that would not trouble ordinary people. This response to items such as dust, foods, food colorings, pollens, molds, or animals is an allergic response. Children with asthma may also develop symptoms after exercise, infection, emotional stress, or a change in the weather.

## RATIONALE FOR TREATMENT

Treatment of asthma is geared to relieving symptoms so that the asthma does not interfere with your child's ability to participate in a full array of physical and social activities. Medications do not cure asthma, but many children will have progressively fewer symptoms or even no symptoms at all as adults. Treatment depends on whether your child's asthma is severe, frequent, chronic, or producing dysfuntion. Some asthmatic attacks will spontaneously resolve, others require only conscious efforts to relax or eliminate an irritant, some require medical intervention.

Our approach to asthma involves three components: (1) avoidance, (2) physical control, and (3) medical treatment.

## HOME TREATMENT

*Avoidance* What should your child avoid? A number of things have been shown to provoke asthma symptoms in the sensitive child. They include tobacco smoke, industrial air pollutants, paints, perfumes, sawdust, insecticides, medications (aspirin, penicillin, erythromycin, tetracycline, neomycin, anesthetics, iron), and allergens. The most common substances (or allergens) that provoke asthma in allergic individuals include pollens (grass, weeds, and trees), molds, animal (especially cat) skins and feathers, insects, food, and dust. Most children sensitive to dust are really allergic to parts of a tiny insect known as a dust mite. This mite can be partly controlled by covering mattresses with plastic. There is an unclear relationship between asthma and common allergenic foods such as grains (wheat), cow's milk, nuts, egg-whites, seafood, legumes, and pork. Avoiding these foods may delay the onset of asthma in some children destined to develop asthma.

Generally, the clues to allergen-provoked asthma are clear. Your child may develop wheezing when petting a cat. Allergic responses other than asthma may develop. Pollens or cats may cause watery, itchy eyes. Children may have asthma only during a particular pollen season. If the responsible agent can be reliably identified you have taken a step forward in learning how to control your child's asthma. However, if you are uncertain, or if your suspicions may jeopardize household harmony by accusing (or removing) a pet, it is possible to have tests performed to identify your child's allergies. These tests (skin or blood tests) can be expensive. Although they are reasonably accurate, several types of test errors may occur. The test may indicate your child is allergic to cats, when this is not really true. The other type of error may exonerate your favorite tree, which may indeed be causing your child's asthma. The tests are only additional supportive evidence; like any other evidence they can be misleading. The best decision about a specific allergy is made by carefully weighing all the evidence you and your child can gather and then looking to skin tests for additional confirmation.

Although identifying and removing a particular pet or plant may be useful, there are some general things you can do to reduce your child's exposure to potential allergens. Because children sleep eight to ten hours daily, they spend most of their time at home in their bedrooms. Cleaning and furnishing this room properly is your best allergen-control strategy. Thick carpeting, felt rug pads, heavy drapes, upholstered furniture, and feather pillows should be avoided. Although is is easy to replace a pillow, it is not always possible to remove carpeting from rented housing. Frequent (at least weekly) vacuuming is needed. Use clean vacuum bags and a well-tuned vacuum cleaner, and make sure that your child is out of the room. Floors and hard surfaces should be washed frequently. Keep closets closed and clutter minimized. Books should be read but stored elsewhere; they collect dust. Only washable stuffed animals should be permitted. Ancient hand-me-down teddy bears may be filled with animal hair or dust commensurate with their age. Time, courage, and patience will allow you to perform home taxidermy; teddy can be eviscerated, washed, and restuffed with foam rubber. Plants should be avoided. Pets should never sleep in the child's room. Even if your child does not have a pet allergy, pollen, dust, and molds can hitch-hike in and on the pet's hair. Finally, heating and air-conditioner filters should be changed regularly. If your child's asthma is severe you should consider purchasing an air purifier. Negative ion generators are useful in eliminating dust for only a small area surrounding the unit.

*Physical Control*   Many factors that cause an asthma attack can be controlled. So far we have discussed allergens. Exercise can also cause breathing difficulties. This is especially true of sports calling for sudden bursts of energy, such as sprinting. Exercise requiring a long, steady amount of energy, such as swimming, bicycling, or jogging, can usually be enjoyed by most asthmatics. Warming up slowly before playing a sport and staying in good physical condition can minimize the wheezing caused by exercise.

Emotions can also aggravate asthma. Extreme anger or excitement will cause some children to have asthma symptoms. If your child's feelings seem to be producing an acute asthma attack, you may be able to help by distracting the child with stories or having your child relax and imagine being in a favorite special place. Children with severe asthma may be helped by receiving special instructions from physicians skilled in techniques of relaxation or self-hypnosis focusing on expanding the airways.

Additional physical relief may be achieved by breathing exercises. Breathing exercises may help in two ways: by helping your child to relax, and by moving air through the lungs more efficiently. The best way to breathe during asthma is sitting in a chair leaning forward. After breathing in, air should be blown out very slowly while counting to five. To help push all the air out your child should use stomach muscles; you can help by pushing your hand against your child's belly to demonstrate how this can help when breathing out.

The final measure you can take before resorting to medication is to encourage drinking plenty of liquids. Keeping well hydrated may prevent thickening of mucus.

## TREATMENT AFTER CONSULTING YOUR PHYSICIAN

Medicines used to treat asthma work against the problems of muscle constriction of the air passages (bronchodilators) and in fighting the inflammation leading to the swelling and mucus (steroids). Other medical approaches are directed toward preventing rather than treating asthma and include the inhalant cromolyn and allergy shots. We will describe each of these four medical approaches.

## TREATMENT WITH MEDICATION

### BRONCHODILATORS

Bronchodilators have been in use for over seventy-five years. They are available in forms for injections, inhalation, and oral consumption.

There are two classes of bronchodilators. Sympathomimetic drugs constitute the first class. Epinephrine (also known as adrenaline), the oldest bronchodilator, is one of the most effective medications. Most asthmatics have had at least one injection of epinephrine. This agent is not effective orally, and though it is available as an inhalant it has no place in asthma management in this form. As an injection it is principally used by physicians to make an initial diagnosis or to treat a severe attack. Some physicians have instructed patients how to give their own epinephrine injections. Because this practice is not widespread, we shall not discuss it here; it is something that can be discussed with your doctor.

Oral bronchodilators in the same class as epinephrine that are also commonly used include metaproterenol sulfate (Alupent), terbutaline sulfate (Brethine, Bricanyl), and ephedrine. Albuterol is the newest medication approved for oral use. Many preparations include fixed combinations of medications that do not allow for proper dosage of each component. Others contain ingredients that are of questionable efficacy in asthma management. We do not recommend fixed-combination drugs for asthma (Asbron G, Brondecon, Bronkolixir, Marax, Quadrinal, Quibron, Tedral, and others).

Bronchodilators available for inhalation include terbutaline sulfate, metaproterenol sulfate (Alupent metered dose inhaler), isoetharine (Bronkometer, Bronkosol), albuterol (Ventolin), and isoproterenol (Isuprel, Medihaler-Iso). In general, inhalant medications are not used in younger children because of difficulty in administration as well as lack of experience in usage. For younger children your physician may prescribe a nebulizer, which will allow administration of these medications at home. Nebulizers are costly, generally over $100. Epinephrine is available over the counter as an inhalant. It has more side effects than newer inhalants; we do not recommend its use.

Common side effects with this class of medicine include temporary anxiety, fast heart rate, and increased blood pressure (epinephrine, ephedrine); muscle tremor (all). The advantage of many of the newer drugs (terbutaline sulfate, albuterol) is that they last longer and have fewer side effects involving faster heart rates and blood pressure elevation. The older sympathomimetic drugs had two types of adrenergic properties: alpha adrenergic effects, which raise the heart rate and blood pressure; and beta adrenergic effects, which open air passages. The newer drugs are mainly beta agents. However, they do cause muscle tremor (shaking). This class is not traditionally the first line of treatment in the United States, whereas it is in some countries such as England. We predict that these newer drugs, because of their effectiveness and relative safety, will become the first line of asthma treatment.

Inhalants are powerful drugs! Their widespread overuse resulted in increased deaths of asthmatics in England in the mid-1960s. They should be used only as recommended by a physician even though some may be obtained without a prescription.

*Theophylline*   The number one medicine used in the treatment and prevention of asthma today belongs to the second major class of drugs that cause bronchodilation. This class also includes caffeine and theobromine, found in chocolate, coffee, tea, and cola drinks.

Theophylline works differently from the bronchodilators already discussed and has a different set of side effects, including nausea, vomiting, increased urination, anxiety, and difficulty sleeping. In an overdose of theophylline the heart's rhythm may become irregular and children may have a seizure.

Theophylline is the first line of defense for asthmatics in two situations. Children who have mild asthma characterized by occasional bouts of wheezing or coughing about three or four times per year can take theophylline at home. Most of these children will respond within a week, and will probably not have severe enough asthma to require a doctor's visit or epinephrine injection.

For those children troubled with more severe asthma—six or more bouts annually, a bout requiring epinephrine in the past six months, an attack causing hospitalization in the past year, or illness requiring school absence of more than six days each semester—daily theophylline may need to be administered to prevent asthma attacks.

Parents can give theophylline in a variety of oral prescription forms; rectal suppositories are not reliable and should be given only in the very rare situation of *extreme* vomiting that persists in the face of normal blood theophylline levels.

Theophylline will prevent the way that phenytoin (Dilantin), a medicine used to treat seizures, is absorbed in the body. If your child is taking erythromycin, theophylline may build up in the body to higher than normal levels. The interactions of these drugs should be discussed by your doctor.

In order to determine your child's precise theophylline needs, your doctor will probably measure blood levels several times. Once requirements are known, a variety of oral preparations, including liquids and tablets, are available. Many products with the same name are available in differing dosages and preparations; when talking on the phone always have the medicine with you. When used as a daily preventive, theophylline is usually dispensed as a long-acting preparation that needs to be taken only twice a day by older children or three times a day by younger children. It is also available as granules that can be sprinkled over food. If theophylline is being used to treat an occasional acute attack it is generally given in a short-acting preparation.

### STEROIDS

When children do not respond to bronchodilators, steroids are the next step in medically reversing the problem of narrowed air passages. Although steroids are very effective in stopping an asthma attack, their many side effects demand judicious use. The most common side effects seen with chronic, prolonged use of steroids include slowing of growth, obesity, diminished ability to fight infection, and ulcers. Fortunately, many years of experience with using steroids have shown how to avoid some complications. For example, growth effects can be avoided by using steroids every other day or by inhalation.

Steroids are used principally in two types of situations. For a moderately severe attack unresponsive to bronchodilators, a one-week course, usually daily prednisone, is given. In patients with severe, recurrent asthma that often does not respond to bronchodilators, steroids can be used preventively. In this situation, steroids are administered orally in an every-other-day regimen, or as a daily inhalant (beclomethasone). Younger children cannot use an inhalant. Older children have an option. Although steroids taken orally every other day do not suppress growth, children may still gain an excessive amount of weight. Inhalants are a better choice for children who have had complications with oral steroids. Although associated with fewer side effects, beclomethasone inhalant is more expensive, more inconvenient (it must be taken three to four times daily), and more complicated to administer. These are trade-offs you should discuss with your child and your physician.

### CROMOLYN

The newest type of medication available for controlling asthma, cromolyn (Intal), cannot stop an asthmatic attack, but it can prevent attacks if taken daily. Because it is an inhalant, it is not for younger children. Although it may not be quite as effective as theophylline as a preventive measure, it has an impressive safety record to date. Almost all the side effects are minor and transient, such as dry mouth or skin irritation.

Children who have problems with theophylline should certainly be given cromolyn if they need preventive treatment. It is the final line of defense before resorting to the more potent and side effect-causing steroids.

## SUMMARY OF ASTHMA TREATMENT

1. Avoid known irritants and allergens.
2. Use sensible physical measures; warm up before exercise, drink plenty of liquids, breathe slowly and forcefully, practice relaxation exercises.
3. Medical treatments
   Mild asthma: Oral theophylline or an inhalant (metaproterenol sulfate, terbutaline sulfate, or albuterol)
   Moderate asthma: Daily theophylline or daily metaproterenol (or albuterol sulfate or terbutaline sulfate)
   Moderate-severe asthma: A combination of drugs used for moderate asthma, e.g., theophylline and metaproterenol sulfate. Add cromolyn as preventive
   Severe asthma: Add beclomethasone inhalant or every-other-day oral steroids to above.

## ALLERGY SHOTS

It is clear that many asthmatic children are allergic to pollen, dust, animals, or food. Often it is impossible to tell if your child does or does not have asthma triggered by an allergy. Children who have hay fever or who obviously wheeze every time that they are exposed to a certain plant, pet, or tree are more likely to be allergic. If you suspect an allergy there are skin tests or blood tests that may indicate (though none can absolutely prove) if your child has asthma caused by an allergy. These tests are usually done only on children over two years old. If these tests suggest an allergic basis for the asthma, and if avoidance and the use of medications still do not keep your child from suffering with severe asthma, allergy shots can be considered.

The allergy shots, also called hyposensitilization, desensitization, or immunotherapy, are probably effective in reducing the effects of allergic asthma caused by pollen and dust; efficacy has not been satisfactorily proved for food or pet allergy. Allergy shots should not be undertaken lightly. Initially injections are required once or twice weekly. Treatment may be either only during a particular pollen season or year-round. Usually allergy shots are given for a minimum of two years. After several years shots can be given as infrequently as once a month, though severely allergic children may require shots more often. Costs vary widely, but the first year will usually cost over $500, often more than $1,000. Yearly cost thereafter will be considerably less.

### ANTIBIOTICS

Bacterial infections can accompany asthma. If your physician suspects a bacterial infection, an antibiotic will be prescribed. However, antibiotics should not be given routinely for every bout of wheezing, because they do not have a role in preventing asthma.

# CHAPTER TWENTY-EIGHT

# Hay Fever *(Allergic Rhinitis)*

## DESCRIPTION

CHILDREN WHO REGULARLY have sneezing, a runny nose, and watery itchy eyes probably experience these symptoms as a result of allergy. An allergic child has an exaggerated response to substances, such as pollen, that cause little or no problem to nonallergic children. Children who have symptoms during pollinating seasons (grasses and trees in spring, ragweed in the summer and fall) have seasonal allergic rhinitis or hay fever. Often, a child will be allergic to a variety of substances including pollens, molds, and animal danders—this is called perennial allergic rhinitis. However, not all children with sneezing and chronic runny noses are allergic some may have vasomotor rhinitis. Because allergies do not cause this type of rhinitis, treatment directed at allergen avoidance or symptomatic relief will not be successful.

Allergic rhinitis is likely if your child seems to have (1) frequent sneezing, (2) a runny nose, (3) dark circles below the eyes, (4) a crease in the nose due to rubbing it frequently, (5) mouth-breathing at night, and (6) a mild sore throat in the morning that disappears after a few minutes. The major problem with allergic rhinitis is that it is uncomfortable and a real nuisance. It often leads to a feeling of fullness in the ears and occasionally may lead to ear and sinus infections.

## RATIONALE FOR TREATMENT

Allergic children inherit their allergic tendencies. However, environmental influences are also involved. The precise role of infection in enhancing allergic response is unknown. There is some evidence that a baby's diet may have the potential to delay the onset of allergic problems in genetically predisposed children. If you have a strong family history of allergy, it may be beneficial to breast-feed to six months or to avoid cow's milk, eggs, beef, and wheat for six months and substitute soy formula.

If you can identify the source of allergic irritation, for example Aunt Suzie's cat, it may be possible to avoid this irritant; more often pollens are responsible and it is difficult to avoid them. Occasionally it may be helpful to remove an offending bush located outside your child's window.

Several chemicals are released whenever your child has allergic rhinitis. Histamine is one of the main culprits. Although the mainstay of allergic therapy is directed toward blocking the effect of histamine, it is important to remember that this approach is seldom completely satisfactory because of the involvement of numerous other chemicals.

Histamine acts by enlarging the blood vessels going to sites such as the nose and eyes and by causing swelling of the lining of the nose. Antihistamine preparations act by competing for the sites that histamine attacks. Thus, antihistamines can prevent histamines from finding a spot to park and do their damage. Therefore they are more effective in preventing the symptoms induced by histamine than they are in reversing these symptoms. They are most effective in curbing the symptoms of runny nose, sneezing, and itching. They are not useful in reversing a swollen blocked nose. Once the nose is swollen and blocked, shrinkage by either local decongestants (nose drops) or oral decongestants is recommended.

### HOME TREATMENT

Dietary possibilities have previously been mentioned. To learn more about avoiding potential allergens, and allergy-proofing your house, see this section in Chapter 27 on Asthma. The mainstay in the treatment of allergic rhinitis is the class of drugs known as antihistamines. While it is desirable to use antihistamines before symptoms occur this is not always possible. If your child is already experiencing symptoms, antihistamines can be given in order to prevent the further development of symptoms. Unfortunately, most antihistamines cause drowsiness. It is therefore important to determine the effect of an antihistamine on your child before allowing him or her to go to school or ride a bicycle. It is impossible to predict in advance how an individual child will respond to an antihistamine. Many children will develop a tolerance for the drowsiness. Because of the capacity of antihistamines to induce drowsiness, it is usually a good idea to try several different preparations in a quest for the medication that will be the most effective and the least bothersome. Your physician can be helpful in making these suggestions. We usually start out with over-the-counter preparations such as chlorpheniramine maleate.

In addition to their capacity to block some of the effects of histamine, antihistamines also have a drying effect on the lining of the nose.

Oral decongestants are often combined with antihistamines to treat children with allergic rhinitis. Although there is a theoretical basis for the use of oral decongestants, in fact the dosage necessary to cause shrinkage of the blood vessels in the nose may also cause mild and transient elevation of blood pressure and increased heart rate. The true efficacy of decongestants is therefore unknown. Some argue for their combination with antihistamines as a way of counteracting the drowsiness that often accompanies the antihistamine. As a general rule, we do not believe that the best way to deal with chemically induced drowsiness is to counteract it with chemically induced stimulation. We feel that you should continue to look for an antihistamine that does not produce drowsiness in your child. Although we are somewhat concerned by all the mild side effects children may experience from the combination drugs used to treat allergic rhinitis, it is important to point out that the widespread usage of these drugs is a testimony to their relative safety. However, you as a parent must determine whether the side effects caused by these medications are more problematic than the symptoms caused by allergic rhinitis.

At this point in time it does not appear that antihistamine or decongestant medications can prevent children with allergic rhinitis from developing the complication of otitis media.

### TREATMENT AFTER CONSULTING YOUR PHYSICIAN

If the antihistamine preparations discussed in the preceding section do not offer relief, and if your child is experiencing considerable discomfort and functional impairment from his or her allergic rhinitis, several medical approaches are available.

Prescription antihistamines such as brompheniramine, diphenhydramine, tripolidine, or pyrabenzamine may be tried alone or in combination with decongestants. Several steroid nose sprays are currently available. They include beclomethasone, betamethasone, and flunisolide. These products have been demonstrated to offer excellent symptomatic relief. The risk of complications that accompany oral steroids are not a major issue if the nasal sprays are used sparingly and cautiously according to your physician's instructions.

If all these treatments have been unsuccessful, allergic hyposensitization therapy is available. Only you can decide, with your child, if your child is experiencing sufficient discomfort and dysfunction to warrant desensitization. Your physician will most likely refer you to an allergist who will take an extensive history and perform a number of skin tests and possibly blood tests to confirm which substances produce allergy in your child. In general, desensitization is more effective in situations where the allergy is seasonal, and restricted to a few identified pollens such as ragweed. Based on these findings a desensitization mixture will be prepared. Children generally require at least four to six months of weekly injections followed by monthly injections for a year or two and periodic booster shots thereafter. The cost is considerable, usually $500 to $1000 the first year, but may be worth consideration if it reduces a considerable amount of misery in a child.

## IS THE TREATMENT WORKING?

Allergic rhinitis is generally a chronic problem. Because of the complex chemical basis for the symptoms, antihistamines can be expected to reduce but not to eliminate the discomfort experienced during a pollen season or other allergen exposure. Desensitization therapy should cause a reduction in seasonal symptoms. However, if the effect is not pronounced this expensive and painful treatment should be discontinued. If all the above treatments are unsuccessful, your child should be examined for another cause for his or her rhinitis.

# CHAPTER TWENTY-NINE

# Pain

## DESCRIPTION

PAIN IS A UNIVERSAL EXPERIENCE. In children it most often accompanies injury, infection, and emotional stress. Many pains are normal responses of the body to unusual loads. For example, belly pain may be the result of gas produced following the rapid consumption of a soft drink, a leg cramp may follow vigorous exercise, chest pain may occur if a child becomes anxious and breathes too rapidly (hyperventilation). The purpose of this chapter will be to help you manage pain of sudden onset. A discussion of individual pain problems—headache, chest pain, abdominal pain, low-back pain, limb pain as well as chronic pain—is beyond the scope of this book, but this subject is dealt with in detail in *Taking Care of Your Child.*

Most parents quickly become experienced managers of pain. It is not your job to eliminate all pain; an anesthetic life is undesirable. Furthermore, pain often serves a useful function. It can pinpoint the site of an infection in an ear, throat, skin, muscle, or bone. It also forces the body to slow down and may thus protect a mild injury in a joint from becoming aggravated through preventing use.

Understanding the significance of pain must involve consideration of the context and setting. A loud protest of severe belly pain immediately following the announcement of bedtime is never convincing. In general, however, sudden onset of severe pain or pain accompanied by a fever will warrant your contacting your physician.

Probably the most common pain situations you will confront is a tearful child holding a recently bruised, battered, or bloodied body part. The remainder of this section will deal with your approach to this common problem.

## RATIONALE FOR TREATMENT

Experiencing pain involves a series of events. When a part of the body is injured, nerves carry an impulse to a part of the brain that is able to experience this sensation. The nerves that receive the pain stimulus may also connect directly with the nerves that will produce an involuntary or reflex withdrawal of the injured part. This is what happens when you withdraw your body quickly from a burn or pinprick. It is also this type of reflex that enables the eyelids to close quickly to avoid oncoming missiles. Some parts of the body, such as fingertips, have numerous nerves capable of carrying pain messages to the brain and are exquisitely sensitive. The back has much fewer nerves, and the nails have none. Body chemicals also play a role in potentiating pain.

Ultimately it is the brain that processes the pain messages sent by the body. The process is sufficiently intricate to have encompassed many scientific careers and filled numerous volumes. In essence, some of us are more sensitive to pain than are others, and each of us copes with pain differently. What is of practical importance is that there are things you can do with your child that may be able to help him or her experience less pain after an injury, and to cope better with that pain.

Whenever cells are injured, as when a muscle receives a crushing blow, a chemical known as prostaglandin begins to be produced by the cell. Prostaglandin has a role in the process of inflammation, which includes pain, swelling, heat, and even the production of redness in the skin. The basis of some pain treatment is to stop the production of prostaglandin by injured cells. Other chemicals manufactured by the body are essentially natural narcotics and can block the way that pain is experienced.

Therapy aimed at stopping pain is sometimes directed to

the site of an injury, as when a local anesthetic such as xylocaine is given to deaden a torn piece of skin so that it can be sewn back in place. Pain can also be stopped by deadening the brain's ability to perceive it. This occurs with the use of hypnosis and certain narcotics. Often a medication will have the ability to block pain both at the site of the injury and at the brain. Aspirin principally acts by blocking damaged cells from producing prostaglandin at the site of the injury, but it also has an effect on a part of the brain known as the hypothalamus. Narcotics primarily dull the sensibility of the brain and also act on the nerve endings at the location of the pain.

### HOME TREATMENT

You play a very important role in how your child will experience a painful injury. Your actions and your demeanor will be far more important initially than any medication.

First, try not to panic. Your four-year-old's fall from a swing may be more of a blow to her ego than to her bottom. Immediate terror on your face may cause an outpouring of anxiety and tears. It may also make your job of assessing the severity of the problem more difficult.

Second, talk to your child before you set about to determine how extensive the injury is. You might try the following:

1. Acknowledge the injury and pain. "You're cut and I'll bet it hurts."

2. Reassure in a calm voice that this is not permanent. "You want it to end, and it will end soon."

3. Do not lie; leave the outcome open. "I'm not sure when it will end but it should be in a few minutes."

4. Distraction helps. "How many minutes do you think it will take to stop—two, three four?" "I'll bet you'd rather be someplace else right now. Where would that be? At Grandma's house? And what would you be doing there?"

5. Crying is okay. "You can cry if it helps. Would something else help?"

6. Link this event to other, happy outcomes. "Remember last month when your brother hurt his ankle and he went to the doctor's office to get it fixed and then we all went to a movie? Well, now you get to go to the doctor."

After these preliminary words of reassurance, you can evaluate the injury and begin management. Again, only general principles will be mentioned here. The evaluation of numerous injuries are covered in *Taking Care of Your Child.* Most profuse bleeding is due to more than just superficial abrasions and will require medical treatment. The scalp may be an exception. It has so many blood vessels that even slight injuries can cause copious bleeding.

For injuries that you believe need evaluation for possible fracture you should immobilize the limb as best you can by limiting movement of the joint above and below the injury.

Most minor trauma can be helped by the three basics of injury management: rest, ice, and protection. Rest and protection are obvious. Ice should be used cautiously only in the first twenty-four hours. Wrap the ice in a towel and use it for only ten minutes at a time.

After the first few hours, pain may still be bothersome enough to prompt the use of medication. One first-line drug is aspirin, which diminishes the pain of inflammation by blocking prostaglandin formation and by having a slight effect on the brain. Acetaminophen is also an effective first-line drug for the relief of pain. It does not inhibit prostaglandin synthesis as much as aspirin and therefore it is not as useful in reducing the inflammation, swelling, and heat. For children who experience stomach pain or wheezing after aspirin use, acetaminophen is the first drug for pain relief.

## TREATMENT AFTER CONSULTING YOUR PHYSICIAN

Occasionally, prescription medication is needed for the relief of the severe pain following a fracture, extensive burns, or other injury. Codeine, a narcotic medication of the class known as opioids, is most often prescribed for these problems. Codeine works primarily by interfering with chemicals carrying the pain impulse between nerves in the brain and in the spinal cord.

Because of its different mechanisms of action, codeine is often combined with aspirin or acetaminophen when additional pain relief is required.

Propoxyphene (Darvon) has not been shown to be as effective as aspirin in pain relief, and we do not recommend it for children.

Nonmedication approaches may be offered by your physician for special situations. Hypnosis, including visual imagery and relaxation techniques, has been effective in relieving acute pain.

### Is the Treatment Working?

Only anesthesia eliminates pain. All the methods described in this chapter act primarily to decrease the sensation of pain. Your support can help your child's reaction to that sensation. An adverse reaction to the painful sensation may cause more suffering than does the sensation itself. If your child is still having difficulty, as evidenced by persistent crying, regression, or inability to sleep, your physician should be notified and a new strategy for use of additional techniques or medication discussed.

### A Guide to Making Decisions When Your Child Has Pain

**See your physician *NOW* for the following symptoms:**

1. Headache associated with any of the following: stiff neck, marked irritability, lethargy, severe pain, visual difficulties, repeated vomiting, purple rash

2. Chest pain that is severe or accompanied by shortness of breath

3. Abdominal pain accompanied by: black or bloody stools, severe pain, recent abdominal injury, bloody vomiting, possible poison or drug ingestion

4. Sore throat accompanied by drooling or shortness of breath

**See your physician *TODAY* for any of the following symptoms:**

1. Earache
2. Sore throat that is severe or has lasted more than several hours
3. Headache associated with fever that is not clearly due to a cold
4. Chest pain accompanied by wheezing, fever, or rapid breathing
5. Abdominal pain lasting more than several hours or combined with: vomiting without bowel movement, vomiting and intermittent pain, pain in one part of the abdomen, yellow jaundice, painful or bloody urination, sore throat, rapid breathing, swollen glands, possible sickle-cell disease, rash, joint pain
6. Pain when urinating
7. Pain in a joint or limb accompanied by fever, swelling, redness, limitation of motion, warmth, rash, abdominal pain, painful urination, leg symptoms

**Make an *APPOINTMENT* with your physician if your child has the following symptoms:**

1. Headache that has lasted more than several days
2. Recurrent head, abdomen, chest, or limb pain causing school absences or problems with friends or family
3. Joint or limb pain lasting more than several days

You may apply **HOME TREATMENT** for these symptoms **only if they are not** accompanied by the characteristics described in this list.

# CHAPTER THIRTY

# Behavioral Problems

CURRENTLY thousands of children in the United States are taking drugs to alter and improve behavior. In one study of a school system in Baltimore County, 2% of the children were taking stimulant medication for hyperactivity. This widespread use of drugs that change behavior (psychoactive drugs) undoubtedly represents inappropriate treatment of a large number of children whose behavior problems are better controlled in other ways. This abuse of psychoactive drugs has stirred considerable outrage and controversy, much of it justified. Unfortunately this controversy has also obscured the fact that carefully selected children may profit greatly from an *appropriate* psychoactive drug. For a child with behavior problems, the use of psychoactive drugs raises several important questions. Does my child absolutely need these drugs? Will my child need them for the rest of his or her life? How harmful or dangerous are these drugs? How will I know if they work? In this chapter we will try to answer these questions, separating where possible what is fact from what is speculation. What we will not do in this chapter is give you criteria for diagnosing behavioral problems in your child. This is a difficult problem for the best of health professionals, and one that cannot be dealt with in a few pages.

Although specific criteria for the use of psychoactive drugs are difficult to determine, there are important guidelines that can assist you in this decision.

1. The use of psychoactive drugs is a serious therapeutic decision. These drugs should be used only for behavioral problems that are sufficiently severe to interfere with your child's ability to function at home, school, or with friends.

2. Psychoactive drugs are rarely indicated as the first or only mode of treatment. Frequently behavior modification, changes in the home environment, special classes in school, or skilled counselling will be sufficient. At least one or some of these treatments should be used concomitantly with psychoactive drugs.

3. When psychoactive drugs are used, their effect should be directed at specific behavior such as increasing attention; these drugs should *not* be used for such diffuse reasons as calming down your child, increasing his or her learning, or improving his or her relationship with friends.

If you and your physician decide that a psychoactive drug may be beneficial for your child, there are several important principles of drug treatment that should be kept in mind.

1. Each child should be treated as an individual, and the use of a psychoactive drug as your own scientific experiment. It will be your observations of your child, and those of his or her physician and teacher, that will determine if a particular medicine is helpful.

2. Treatment with psychoactive drugs should not be viewed as a life-long commitment. There should be periods when your child is without drugs. This can occur as frequently as every weekend or as infrequently as once every two years.

3. Close supervision of drug treatment is imperative. Weekly assessment in the beginning can be done by phone with the school and with you. Once the proper dosage of medication is established your child should be examined at least every six months to evaluate possible side effects. All serious side effects should be reported as they occur.

4. Drug treatment should always be undertaken as part of a comprehensive treatment plan that should include educational and environmental manipulations, and possibly counseling. Drugs should *never* be prescribed as the only mode of treatment.

## COMMON DISORDERS TREATED
## WITH PSYCHOACTIVE DRUGS

### "HYPERACTIVE" CHILDREN: ATTENTION DEFICIT DISORDER

Mild cases of hyperactivity or attentional deficit will usually respond to increased precision and structure at home, appropriate educational interventions in the school, and the use of behavioral management techniques by parents and teachers. For those children for whom these interventions are insufficient, a trial of psychoactive drugs may be warranted. Stimulant medications have been the most frequently employed class of drugs for this disorder. There are no absolutely reliable markers that distinguish children who will respond favorably from those who will not respond. Past experience with stimulant medications has shown that roughly 75% of children will respond favorably to the treatment. Your physician cannot predict in advance whether or not your child will respond to stimulant medication. There have been a number of behavioral ratings scales employed in the past to predict which child will respond to medication, but in spite of claims of success these tests have not been able to consistently predict drug response.

For this reason a trial of medication may be the only way of determining if a behavior problem that will respond to these medications is present. This diagnostic-therapeutic trial must be approached with caution. Many children will respond initially with increased attention span and alertness. This reaction may be related to the actions of the drug or it may be due to a placebo effect. The medication should improve your child's ability to function in important areas. In order to document this improvement, you need to define areas of dysfunction in advance, in a way that is clearly understandable to you, to your child, and to your physician. An example of this degree of definition would be taking a complaint such as "John can't sit down and do his homework" and redefining it as (1) he cannot begin his homework when asked, (2) he cannot stay at one assignment for more than five minutes, and (3) he cannot finish his homework after it has been started. By breaking this initial complaint down into easily understandable components it is easier to assess the effect of the medication on specific components of the problem. It is your assessment, combined with the teacher's assessment, that will provide the most reliable information as to the effectiveness of the medication.

## BEDWETTING (NOCTURNAL ENURESIS)

Bedwetting is a common problem that is frequently treated with a psychoactive drug, imipramine (Tofranil). Enuresis is not a behavioral disorder; it is rather a problem of maturation. Virtually all enuresis will disappear if you wait until your child's adolescence. However, if the enuresis is severely affecting your child's life, imipramine may have a role in alleviating the problem. For a more detailed discussion of enuresis, see Chapter 25.

## ANXIETY AND DEPRESSION

Anxious, depressed, or unhappy children are best treated with counseling and, when necessary, psychotherapy. There is rarely, if ever, a need for antianxiety medicines (e.g., diazepam or Valium). The use of antidepressants in severely depressed children is controversial; if these medications are used it should be by a child psychiatrist with experience in using psychoactive drugs in children. The area, however, is sufficiently controversial that a second opinion should be sought before using antianxiety or antidepressant medications for behavioral disorders in children.

## INSOMNIA

Insomnia is a common but not too serious problem in children. It may be related to stress, anxiety, a sleep-wake cycle that is out of synchrony with bedtime (e.g., jet lag), or too much stimulation near bedtime. If the insomnia becomes severe or diabling, counseling should be sought from a mental health professional. Sleeping medications are rarely indicated in children. If they are given, it should be under the guidance of an experienced child psychiatrist. There are some types of sleep problems, such as sleep walking or night terrors* that may require mild tranquilizers such as diazepam (Valium) to alleviate the problem.

## SPECIFIC PSYCHOACTIVE DRUGS
### STIMULANTS USED FOR ATTENTION DEFICIT DISORDER

*Methylphenidate (Ritalin)*  Methylphenidate is given before breakfast and, if the effects appear to wear off in the afternoon, again at lunch. The medicine is begun at a dosage of 5 mg and increased until either the desired effects are achieved or there are some signs of toxicity. Finding the correct dose is important and unfortunately sometimes difficult. Some experts feel that methylphenidate at a given dose improves learning abilities, but requires a higher dose to effect an improvement in social behavior. What really complicates the situation is that when the higher doses required to change social behavior are used there may be deterioration in learning ability. The dose of methylphenidate may have to be titrated to achieve a specific effect on either learning ability or social behavior. Close cooperation is required between you and your physician to arrive at the proper dose for the maximum therapeutic effect. The maximal dose employed by most experts is 60 mg per day. If no effect on specific behavior is observed after one month at this dosage, the drug should be discontinued. The most commonly observed side effects of methylphenidate are loss of appetite and insomnia. These symptoms usually occur during the first several weeks of therapy and tend to diminish as tolerance develops. Loss of appetite can be minimized by giving the drug with meals, and insomnia can be avoided by restricting drug administration to morning hours.

A great deal of publicity has been given to suppression of growth with the chronic administration of methylphenidate. Some investigators have reported a decrease in growth proportional to the amount and duration of treatment. Interestingly, when stimulant medications were discontinued in

---

*Night terrors are different from nightmares. With night terrors your child is awake and incoherent, and cannot remember the experience in the morning.

these children, their growth rebounded to normal in a matter of months. It is also important to note that several investigators have refuted the claim that methylphenidate causes any significant growth retardation at all. The final answer is not known with respect to growth suppression. Your child, however, should have his growth closely monitored, and if growth suppression occurs, you will have to weigh the costs and benefits of discontinuing the medication. Additional side effects can include headaches, abdominal pain, dizziness, anxiety, palpitations, constipation, rashes, nightmare, dry mouth, and high blood pressure.

What about the long-term effects of methylphenidate? In spite of the long list of possible short-term side effects there have been no serious long-term side effects reported on the heart, blood pressure, or other organs of the body. There has been no documented predisposition to drug abuse later in life. On the other side of the coin, there have been few documented long-term benefits of stimulant drug treatment. Although the short-term effects are frequently dramatic, there is little evidence to support any long-term effects of stimulant drug treatment on either social or learning behavior. Some investigations have even suggested that children on stimulant drugs are subject to state-dependent learning, i.e., the child will retain what is learned while on the drug only as long as the drug is continued. This research is controversial, but it does underscore the problem for the parent and physician alike in determining what are the long-term risks and benefits of stimulant medication.

*Dextroamphetamine (Dexedrine)* Dextroamphetamine is similar in its actions and side effects to methylphenidate. It is begun at a dose of 2–5 mg and can be gradually increased until the desired effects are achieved or a maximal dose of 40 mg per day is reached. Information on whether different doses of dextroamphetamine achieve different effects with respect to social and learning behavior is not available. Dexedrine, however, does have greater appetite suppressant effects, and is also reported to cause greater growth suppression than methylphenidate. This phenomenon is reversible after the drug is discontinued. The remainder of the side effects are similar to those listed for methylphenidate. There is greater experience with this drug in children aged three to six years, and dextroamphetamine is the drug of choice for this age group.

*Pemoline (Cylert)* Pemoline is the third stimulant commonly employed. It has the advantage of a longer duration of action and may be given once a day in the morning. The usual starting dose is 18.75 mg, which may be increased to 37.5 or 75 mg until either the desired effect or side effects are observed. The side effects associated with pemoline are similar to those found with methylprenidate and dextroamphetamine, with insomnia and loss of appetite leading the list. Growth suppression has not been well documented for pemoline. There have however been several cases of mild liver damage in some patients, the long-term significance of which is not known.

*Caffeine* For the past several years there have been reports from parents and physicians that hyperactive children who drank coffee showed improvement in their attention spans. Research done to confirm these impressions has been contradictory at best, with studies showing improvement, no improvement, and even worsening of symptoms.

## Major Tranquilizers

As previously mentioned, there is little if any role at all for this class of medicine in the treatment of behavioral disorders in children. Rarely, a child with a severe behavioral disturbance will be given one of these drugs under the guidance of a child psychiatrist.

## Minor Tranquilizers

There is little or no indication for the use of these medicines in pediatrics. Counseling and psychotherapy are the preferred alternatives to these drugs.

## ANTIDEPRESSANTS

Imipramine (Tofranil) is the only antidepressant used in pediatrics. This medicine is used not because of its effect on behavior, but rather because of its effect on the bladder and sleep cycle in the treatment of bedwetting. Its use for bedwetting is not recommended under the age of six years. It is given one hour before bedtime, starting in doses as low as 10 mg and increasing up to 100 mg in the older child and adolescent. Minor side effects are changes in behavior, drowsiness, loss of appetite, and dizziness. More serious side effects include damage to the blood, seizures, damage to the heart, and stomach upset. Again, it must be remembered that imipramine is a very dangerous drug, with as little as 500 mg being lethal in small children. Imipramine for enuresis should, in most cases, be prescribed for a three-to-six-month period and then discontinued for a trial period. Imipramine is rarely indicated for the treatment of childhood depression or behavioral disorders.

## ANTIHISTAMINES

Antihistmines have been frequently used to treat insomnia, hyperactivity, and a variety of behavior disorders. Whereas their sedative action is well known to physicians and parents, the chronic use of these drugs in insomnia will not only disturb the sleep cycle but may mask the causes of the insomnia. There have been no good clinical studies to support the use of antihistamines in hyperactivity or in other behavioral disorders; because of this, we cannot recommend their use in these situations.

The side effects of antihistamines are discussed in detail in the chapter on colds.

## HYPNOTICS AND SEDATIVES (SLEEPING PILLS AND POTIONS)

It is not unusual for children with hyperactivity, or other behavioral disorders, to have difficulty falling asleep. Although chronic use of sleeping medicines is to be condemned, some physicians recommend their occasional use. Antihistamines are frequently employed as sleeping medicines and are fairly effective in this capacity with minimal side effects. Another commonly used sleeping medicine is chloral hydrate. In doses of 500 to 1000 mg this is an effective medicine with minimal side effects. The primary approach to insomnia in your child, however, should be through counseling and not medication. Sleeping medicines, if used at all, should be reserved for only exceptional situations, and only with the advice of your physician.

# CHAPTER THIRTY-ONE

# Seizures

By Nancy Humphress Curtis, M.D.*

### DESCRIPTION

A SEIZURE, also known as a convulsion, is not an uncommon occurrence in children. Approximately 3% of young children have a seizure associated with high fever at some time. A child who repeatedly has seizures with or without fever is said to have *epilepsy* or a *seizure disorder*. Epilepsy affects about 1% of the childhood population. Having a seizure does not necessarily mean that a child has epilepsy.

If your child has a seizure for the first time, you should see a physician as soon as possible. A seizure may be the symptom of an underlying problem such as serious infection. Your doctor is the best source of information about the problem. Information travels within the brain and through the nerves to the body in the form of electrical currents. A seizure occurs if the electrical messages suddenly become disorganized and spread abnormally. This causes the outward signs of the seizure.

There are several common types. *Generalized major motor seizures (grand mal)* are usually a frightening experience for a parent to observe. There is a sudden loss of consciousness and sometimes the child's eyes will roll back in the head. The body stiffens forcefully and rhythmic jerking of the muscles may follow. Occasionally only one arm or leg may jerk. After the attack the child is commonly confused and tired. Recurrent seizures without fever are usually major motor seizures. Febrile seizures or fever fits are usually also of this type. Typically a febrile seizure occurs in a child

* Fellow, Division of General Pediatrics, University of California, San Francisco, California.

between six months and five years of age. *Absence attacks
(petit mal)* are most commonly seen in a child between three
and thirteen years of age. The seizure lasts for only five to
fifteen seconds. During that time the child stares vacantly
into space. No jerking occurs, and the episode is often unno-
ticed. Immediately after the seizure the child resumes normal activity, unaware that the seizure has occurred. *Psychomotor (temporal lobe) seizures* are unusual in children less
than ten years old. The attack may begin with an unusual
sensation, such as nausea or abdominal pain. The child may
then stare and be unable to respond when spoken to, perhaps picking at his or her clothes or repeating nonsense
phrases. After the spell the child may be tired or confused.
Sometimes a psychomotor seizure may generalize into a major motor seizure.

### RATIONALE FOR TREATMENT

If your child has had a single febrile seizure, your doctor
may not advise treatment with anticonvulsive medicines because the majority of children who have had a simple febrile
seizure will never have another. However, in certain circumstances a doctor may recommend continuous anticonvulsive
therapy to prevent future febrile seizures. The medication is
effective for this purpose, but there is no evidence that preventing short febrile seizures will reduce the very slight risk
of developing epilepsy at a later time.

The medical reasons to prevent recurrent seizures include
avoiding physical injury from falling during a seizure, and
avoiding the small risk of choking during the attack. A few
people who are untreated or who take their medicines errati-
cally develop a series of prolonged seizures without gaining
consciousness between attacks. This serious condition is
called *status epilepticus.*

There is evidence that it is beneficial to control a child's
seizure disorder early so that the child will be less likely to
have a seizure if the medication is discontinued at a later
time.

Important social reasons to prevent further seizures include the consideration that a child is likely to be labeled "different" if he or she has a seizure in the presence of other children. That is obviously a difficult burden for a child. Additionally, an adolescent cannot obtain his or her automobile driver's license unless these seizures are very reliably controlled.

### HOME TREATMENT

If your child has a seizure at home, take care that he or she is safe from hitting head, arms, and legs against surrounding objects. If your child has a clenched jaw, do not attempt to force an object into the mouth. Stay with your child until the episode is over.

You should treat your child for fever (see Chapter 8) if she or he has had a febrile seizure in the past. You cannot always prevent a recurrent febrile seizure this way, but the odds are in your favor that your child will not have another seizure.

### TREATMENT AFTER CONSULTING YOUR PHYSICIAN

A drug is chosen by its effectiveness and prevention of a particular kind of seizure and for its safety for use in children. Initially a single drug is prescribed. The drug dosage is gradually increased until good seizure control is obtained. The maximum dosage of a drug is limited by the side effects of the medication.

Three of the most commonly used anticonvulsants in this country are phenobarbital, phenytoin, and ethosuximide. Phenobarbital is widely used in children because of its effectiveness, relative safety, and low cost. It is used to prevent recurrent febrile seizures, major motor seizures, and psychomotor attacks. Customarily, phenobarbital is given in doses of 3–5 mg/kg/day. Many physicians advise giving the medicine twice during the day to ensure relatively constant blood levels. However, the entire dosage may be given once a day, usually at bedtime. It may take two or three weeks before the medicine reaches a stable level in the blood.

The most common side effects of phenobarbital are sedation and hyperactivity (overactivity with a very short attention span). Occasionally a child will develop muscular incoordination.

The sedation effects of phenobarbital generally improve or disappear as the child becomes accustomed to the drug. This takes place over a period of several weeks. Overactivity and other behavior disorders such as irritability and insomnia are not uncommon side effects. They may not appear until your child has been taking the medicine for several months. It is more likely to be a problem if your child has had similar problems before beginning the medicine. If the symptoms are a result of the medicine, they usually improve after the drug is discontinued.

Phenytoin is effective for treatment of major motor and psychomotor seizures. It is not helpful for prevention of febrile or petit mal seizures. Phenytoin may be given once daily to adults but it is better to use divided doses for children. Again, this is to ensure relatively constant levels of the medicine in the blood. The average dose of phenytoin is 4–7 mg/kg/day. A stable blood level is achieved over one to two weeks. If there is a pressing need to obtain the therapeutic level more quickly, your doctor may prescribe a higher dose at more frequent intervals over the first day of treatment. This is referred to as a loading dose. A great number of children who take phenytoin develop overgrowth of the gums, which may be minimized by very good oral hygiene and gum massage. Overgrowth of hair may develop on the face, arms, and trunk. Approximately 2–5% of children beginning this drug develop fever, rash, and enlargement of the lymph glands. Other common effects of this medicine are eye-jerking and muscular incoordination that causes staggering, slowed speech, and double vision. You should contact your child's physician if you notice any of these side effects because the medication may need to be adjusted.

Ethosuximide is currently considered the best drug for petit mal seizures. If your child has any other type of seizure as well, an additional anticonvulsant may be needed. This medicine is begun at a low dose (usually 20 mg/kg/day or 250 mg twice a day) and is increased slowly. A stable blood level is attained after about a week on a given dose. Nausea, vomiting, and a decreased appetite are the most common dose-related side effects of this drug. Drowsiness, dizziness, and hiccups are also reported. In high doses a child may have trouble sleeping, or may become agitated.

## Is the Treatment Working?

If the treatment is working well, your child's seizures should be controlled and the medicine should be well tolerated. The amount of medication required varies from one child to another. Similarly, a child's dose may change as she or he grows. Sometimes, measuring the level of the drug in the blood on a given dosage helps to determine the amount of medication needed.

If the seizures are not well controlled despite adequate amounts of one medication your doctor may consider adding a second anticonvulsant drug. Sometimes it is possible to gradually discontinue the use of the first drug if the second drug works well. Whenever your doctor advises changing your child's medication you should be aware of the possible side effects. You may also want to keep a log of the seizures to help assess how well the medication is working.

A common question is when to discontinue medication. Certainly it is possible that after a prolonged period without a seizure (usually two to four years) your doctor will consider gradually stopping your child's medication. Many factors must be considered when making this decision, such as the type of seizures your child has had, how quickly seizure control was achieved, and whether the physical examination is normal. A key point is that the drug must be tapered over a long period of time (weeks to months), because suddenly stopping an anticonvulsant drug may increase the frequency of seizures or may even precipitate status epilepticus.

# CHAPTER THIRTY-TWO

# The "Childhood" Diseases: *Chicken Pox, Mumps, and Measles*

## DESCRIPTION

ENCOUNTERS WITH the childhood diseases used to be an expected part of growing up. Unfortunately not all children survived the encounter—measles can be quite severe and can lead to serious complications including encephalitis and death. But today, measles is fortunately a preventable disease. The immunization is discussed in Chapter 14. Measles, along with mumps, chicken pox, and German measles (rubella), are all caused by viruses. Because there are no medicines effective against viruses the approach to these diseases is to either prevent them through immunizations or treat the symptoms such as pain (Chapter 29), fever (Chapter 15), or rash (Chapter 26). Immunizations are available against mumps and rubella as well as for measles (see Chapter 14). Whereas rubella poses risks to the unborn fetus of a pregnant woman who contracts this infection, it causes virtually no symptoms in children other than a mild rash, a low-grade fever that rarely exceeds 101°F (38.3°C), and occasional joint pains in older children and adolescents. Because rubella so seldom is even detected or requires treatment, we shall confine our discussion to chicken pox, which is quite common and which is not routinely prevented by immunization, and to mumps and measles, which are rapidly disappearing in children who have been properly immunized.

### RATIONALE FOR TREATMENT

Once a diagnosis is made, treatment is always geared to relieving symptoms. If your child has measles or mumps you should check your other children's immunization records and inform parents of playmates. It is possible to prevent or ameliorate these illnesses in contacts by immediate immunization or administration of special immune globulin. Children who were immunized against measles at twelve months or less may not be fully protected and should be reimmunized. It is impossible to prevent complications of measles such as pneumonia, hemorrhages, skin rash, or encephalitis once the illness is established.

### HOME TREATMENT

*Chicken Pox*   Chicken pox is the mildest childhood disease and usually causes only annoying symptoms. Generally there are no symptoms before the rash appears, but occasionally there may be some fatigue or mild fever on the day before the rash is noted. The typical rash appears in several stages including flat red splotches, tiny pimple-like bumps, fluid-filled blisters called vesicles, and crusted sores. Your child is contagious until the sores have finished crusting. Keep your child away from any other children who may be taking steroids (asthmatics) or children with cancer or immune problems.

The major symptoms that require treatment include fever and the itchiness of the rash. Fever in chicken pox should *not* be treated with aspirin because of the slightly increased chance that the child with chicken pox who is given aspirin may develop a rare complication known as Reye's syndrome (coma, brain swelling, and swollen liver). Therefore fever should be treated with acetaminophen and other measures recommended in the section on fever (Chapter 15).

To prevent the scarring that can result from scratching the chicken pox vesicles, be sure to cut your child's fingernails and wash the hands frequently. The skin should be kept clean with soap and water. Vesicles may appear in the mouth and may be helped with salt-water gargles (one-half teaspoon salt to an eight-ounce glass of water).

To reduce the itching, which is often quite annoying, we recommend several approaches. Cooling generally reduces itching. Cooling can be accomplished with cool baths, or simply by wetting the skin and allowing cooling to occur during the process of water evaporation. Shake lotions such as calamine lotion contain zinc oxide, which is soothing, and water, which will evaporate and cool. Do not use any lotion with an antihistamine, which can irritate the skin. A warm bath will intensify the itching during the bathing period but will provide several hours of markedly reduced itching following the bath.

*Mumps*  Mumps is a viral infection involving the salivary glands. These main glands are located directly below and in front of the ear. The glands swell and are quite painful. Foods that cause an outpouring of saliva (such as lemons, oranges, or pickles) may make the pain worse. The pain and fever can be reduced with either acetaminophen or aspirin. Although eating may be difficult, it is important to maintain adequate fluid intake. Avoid citrus fruits.

*Measles*  Children with measles are generally moderately ill. They usually have a fever, an extensive rash, a brassy cough, and conjunctivitis. The fever can be reduced with acetaminophen or aspirin. Unlike the rash of chicken pox, measles is usually a confluent rash covering nearly the entire torso and extending to the face and extremities as well. Fortunately it is usually not itchy and requires no specific treatment. The cough may be helped by a vaporizer. Dim lighting in the room often makes the child feel more comfortable because of the eyes' sensitivity to light.

### TREATMENT AFTER CONSULTING YOUR PHYSICIAN

Your physician can offer little in the management of these viral diseases unless a bacterial complication such as otitis or pneumonia occurs (measles). To help relieve itching of chicken pox, antihistamines (such as hydroxyzine, cyproheptadine, and diphenhydramine hydrochloride) may be prescribed. We recommend their usage only if the anti-itch remedies suggested here have failed.

## IS THE TREATMENT WORKING?

Your children's reports are the best guide for the symptoms of itching and pain. All these illnesses will run their course. Measles lasts seven to ten days. Mumps usually lasts a week. Although chicken pox is usually mild, new crops of vesicles often occur for eight to nine days, and crusting may not be completed for nine to thirteen days.

# Part IV

# COMMONLY USED MEDICINES

# How to Use This Section

Each medication discussion is intended to provide information for you to use as a guide. Your physician may have a good reason for using a medication differently. If you have any concern about the proper usage of a medication, always check with your physician and/or pharamcist.

Discussions are organized as follows.

## Name

Usually the generic name, except where noted as in combination drugs. The manufacturer's name accompanies each brand name as a main heading.

*Brand Names:* Commonly available products

*Description and Uses:* The principal ways in which the medication is used.

*Preparations: Types of preparations:*

*Tablets* and *capsules* are both oral preparations which, in general, must be swallowed. Some capusles are *enteric coated* or designed to dissolve in the intestines thus sparing the stomach the irritating effects of medicine. With certain capsules (e.g. Slo-Phyllin) you may open the clear capsule and mix the medicine-containing granules in food.

Liquid preparations include *elixirs,* which contain alcohol, as well as *syrups,* which contain sugar and *aromatic waters* which are solutions of water with oil, such as peppermint.

*Drops* of a given preparation are generally more concentrated than other liquid forms.

Topical preparations include lotions which are predominantly a water vehicle; *creams* which are usually white and a combination of oil-in-water and are only fair lubricants; *ointments* which are usually gray, excellent lubricants, and a combination of water-in-oil. *Oils* are substances such as mineral oil, petrolatum, or lanolin. *Gels* are usually clear and contain water, alcohol, and glycols.

*Dosage:* Caution. This is an approximate guide. Children vary considerably in both size and medication requirements. In calculating dosages we use the following weights: infants = 5 kg or 11 pounds, toddlers = 10 kg or 22 pounds, school-age children = 20 kg or 45 pounds, adolescents = 50 kg or 110 pounds. If your child's dosage is considerably more or less, you should check with your physician or pharmacist.

*Side Effects:* Each side effect is listed in terms of relative frequency. In general, common side effects occur in more than 1% of cases. Infrequent side effects are usually found in between 1 out of 100 and 1 out of 1000 persons taking the medicine. Rare side effects occur much less often. In general, for side effects labeled with one star you may continue giving the medicine unless the symptom becomes particularly troublesome, in which case you should contact your physician. For two-star side effects you should contact your physician but may continue with the medicine. Three-star side effects require that you promptly stop the medicine and contact your physician.

*Comments:* Unless otherwise stated in this section, you may assume that preparations can be stored at room temperature. Always make sure that caps are tightly in place and that medications cannot be reached by small children.* Other important issues, specific to an individual medication, will be discussed here.

---

* Always note the expiration date on the bottle or tube. Do not use the medicine after expiration date. These bottles should be thrown out.

# Alphabetical Descriptions of Medications

## Acetaminophen

*Brand Names:*  Datril, Liquiprin, Phenaphen, Tempra, Tylenol

*Description and Uses:*  Acetaminophen is as effective as aspirin in reducing fever and pain. It is not as good an anti-inflammatory agent, but this is of no consequence for its ordinary use in children. It is preferred over aspirin because it has fewer side effects and is less toxic. It is also available in liquid preparations, making it easier to administer to infants.

*Preparations:*  (Tylenol) Drops: 80 mg/0.8 cc, 60 mg/10.6 cc. Elixir: 160 mg/5 cc, 120 mg/5 cc. Tablets: 81 mg/chewable tablet

*Dosage:*  INFANTS: 40 mg every 4 to 6 hours
TODDLERS: 120 mg every 4 to 6 hours
SCHOOL AGE: 240 mg every 4 to 6 hours
ADOLESCENTS: 480 mg every 4 to 6 hours

Acetaminophen can be combined with aspirin to reduce fever and given every 6 hours.

*Side Effects:*  RARE: Dizziness,** drowsiness**

In occasional overdoses yellowing of eyes and skin (liver damage) can occur.

*Comments:* Be careful with liquid dosages. The drops are 4 times the strength of the elixir.

## Acetic Acid Ear Solution

*Brand Names:* Orlex Otic, Otic Domeboro Solution, and VōSol Otic

*Description and Uses:* These solutions are useful in treating external otitis media (including swimmer's ear). They are effective against common types of infecting bacteria and fungi. They also relieve swelling and consequently may reduce the associated pain. These preparations have advantages over many antibiotic drops, which may cause sensitization or influence the emergence of resistant bacteria or create an overgrowth of other bacteria. A comparable solution may be made at home by mixing equal parts of white vinegar (5%) and water.

*Preparations:* Orlex Otic Solution: 2% acetic acid with 0.1% chlorometa-xylenol and propylene glycol. VōSol Otic Solution: 2% acetic acid with propylene glycol and 3% propylene glycol diacetate. Otic Domeboro Solution: 2% acetic acid in aluminum acetate

*Dosage:* For the first day a cotton wick is placed in the affected ear and saturated with solution. It is removed the next day and 3 to 4 drops are instilled in the ear 3 to 4 times daily.

*Side Effects:* INFREQUENT: Irritation or stinging of ear canal**

*Comments:* When swelling is severe the above agents may be combined with a steroid, 1% cortisol, to reduce swelling and inflammation. These preparations are VōSol HC, Orlex HC Otic. Do not use these preparations in children with chicken pox.

Many ear preparations are available with the antibiotic neomycin. This antibiotic is sensitizing and can cause skin reactions. In addition, there is the potential for middle-ear toxicity with the drug; if a middle-ear perforation exists, we do not recommend its use.

## Acne Preparations (Other than Benzoyl Peroxide or Retinoic Acid)

*Brand Names:* Acne-Dome, Acnomel, Exzit, Fomac, Keralyt, phisoAc

*Description and Uses:* The following classes of agents may be found in preparations designed to combat acne: Peeling agents: Sulfur, resorcinol, salicylic acid. Antiseptics: Phenol, parachlorometaxylenol, providone-iodine, sodium sulfacetamide, clioquinol. Drying agents: Alcohol, zinc compounds, sodium thiosulfate. Abrasives: Aluminum oxide. Although peeling agents may be effective, two currently available prescriptions, benzoyl peroxide and tretinoin, have known efficacy against acne. Abrasives may cause problems if used with these two effective drugs.

*Preparations:* Soaps, cleansers, lotions, gels, creams

*Dosage:* Varies with product. Usually applied 1 to 3 times daily

*Side Effects:* Potential skin irritation

*Comments:* These agents are not as effective as benzoyl peroxide or tretinoin. Only sulfur or resorcinol have a possible role in patients sensitive to more effective products.

## Actifed

*Combination Drug:* Pseudoephedrine, Tripolidine

*Description and Uses:* A combination of an antihistamine and an adrenergic drug. These drugs both have activities that have a drying effect on the nasal lining. They each have opposite side effects (drowsiness and restlessness) but should not be combined in order to balance these undesirable symptoms. This preparation may be useful for symptomatic relief of colds. There is no evidence that it is efficacious for preventing or treating otitis media.

*Preparations:* Tablet: 2.5 mg tripolidine and 60 mg pseudoephedrine. Syrup: 1.25 mg tripolidine and 30 mg pseudoephedrine/5 ml

*Dosage:*  INFANTS: ½ teaspoon three times daily
TODDLERS: 1 teaspoon three times daily
SCHOOL AGE: 2 teaspoons or 1 tablet three times daily
ADOLESCENTS: 2–3 teaspoons or 1–1½ tablets

*Side Effects:*  See tripolidine, pseudoephedrine

## Albuterol

*Brand Names:*  Proventil, Ventolin

*Description and Uses:*  Albuterol is a newer adrenergic drug with good selectivity for relaxing bronchial muscles to relieve asthma attacks but without much of the cardiac stimulant effects of older, less selective adrenergic drugs such as isoproterenol and ephedrine.

*Preparations:*  Currently available as a metered-dose aerosol unit for oral inhalation and 2 and 4 mg tablets

*Dosage:* Safety and effectiveness in children less than twelve years old has not been established. School-age children (over twelve years old) and adolescents: 2 inhalations every 4 to 6 hours. The proper use of an inhalant requires practice. The aerosol-inhaler unit must be shaken immediately before each use. Your child must learn to breathe out fully and then press the top of the aerosol while breathing in deeply. Your child should then hold his or her breath as long as possible. The above sequence can be repeated for a second inhalation after waiting one minute. The oral preparation is given 2–4 mg every 6–8 hours (start at 2 mg and gradually increase dose to minimize side effects).

*Side Effects:*   As with other aerosols, inhaling albuterol may worsen the bronchospasm of asthma. The drug should be immediately stopped and your physician notified.

> COMMON: Nausea***
>
> INFREQUENT: Dry throat,* palpitations,*** increased heart rate,*** muscle tremor,*** vomiting,*** nervousness,*** bad taste***

*Comments:*   Albuterol is the newest selective adrenergic drug to be released as an aerosol. It is an acceptable alternative to metaproterenol aerosol although currently more expensive. It is preferable to isoproterenol and epinephrine inhalants because it has fewer undesirable cardiac effects. Contents of the aerosolized cannister are under pressure. Therefore, exercise the usual caution with such a container; avoid puncturing or exposure to any temperature above 120°F.

## Aluminum Acetate Solution (Burow's Solution)

*Brand Names:*   Other wet dressings include Bluboro and Domeboro (calcium acetate and aluminum sulfate) and AluWets (aluminum chloride hexahydrate)

*Description and Uses:*   Aluminum acetate 5% solution can be diluted with 10 to 40 parts of water to provide an effective wet dressing. Wet dressings are often recommended for acute skin problems with crusting and oozing lesions. The water in the dressing cools, soothes, cleanses, and helps combat the inflammatory process.

*Preparation:*   5% solution

*Dosage:*   Dilute 1 part Burow's solution with 10 to 40 parts water. Apply on skin. *Do not cover with plastic or rubber.* Change dressing every 5 to 15 minutes for up to 8 changes in 2 hours.

*Side Effects:*   Can irritate skin if not diluted

*Comments:*   Other wet dressings are not as satisfactory as Burow's solution. Potassium permanganate and silver nitrate both stain skin or clothing and are more irritating. Silver nitrate has more antibacterial properties.

## Amoxicillin

*Brand Names:*   Amoxil, Polymox, Robamox, Sumox, Trimox, Utimox, Wymox

*Description and Uses:*   Amoxicillin is an antibiotic very closely related to ampicillin. It is used for the same conditions as ampicillin, except that it is not used for treating bacterial diarrhea. Several studies have suggested that amoxicillin may have slightly fewer side effects, such as the fine rash and diarrhea seen commonly with ampicillin. However, we feel that these studies are inconclusive. Amoxicillin's advantage over ampicillin is that it need be given only 3 times a day instead of 4. However, it is still slightly more expensive than ampicillin for a treatment course.

*Preparations:*   Suspension: 125mg/5ml, 250 mg/5ml. Capsules: 250, 500 mg

*Dosage:*   INFANTS: 62.5 mg 3 times per day
TODDLERS: 125 mg 3 times per day
SCHOOL AGE: 250 mg 3 times per day
ADOLESCENTS: 250 mg 3 times per day

*Storage:*   Suspension should be refrigerated

*Side Effects:*   COMMON: Diarrhea,** yeast infection—mouth or diaper area,** rash, fine bumps, red itchy—onset third day**
RARE: Hives—red, blotchy, itchy rash—onset immediately***
SERIOUS ALLERGIC REACTION: Trouble breathing, dizzy, faint, pale***

*Comments:* Amoxicillin is frequently favored over ampicillin for treatment of infections because it may cause less diarrhea. This has not been well proven. Amoxicillin has an additional advantage over ampicillin in that it may be given 3 instead of 4 times a day. It should not be given to children with a known allergy to penicillin. It may be taken with meals.

## Ampicillin

*Brand Names:* Amcill, D-Amp, Divercillin, Omnipen, Pen-A, Penbriten, Pensyn, Polycillin, Principen, Saramp, SK-Ampicillin, Supen, Totacillin

*Description and Uses:* Ampicillin is an antibiotic related to penicillin that is effective in killing a wide variety of bacteria that commonly cause infections in children. For many years it has been the first-line drug for treating otitis media in children. In some parts of the country, *Hemophilus influenzae*, a bacterium responsible for many cases of otitis media, is developing resistance to ampicillin and physicians may use other, costlier drugs as an initial treatment. Ampicillin is also useful in treating urinary tract infections. Several studies have suggested that a 1- to 3-day course is sufficient to treat an uncomplicated lower-urinary infection. Ampicillin is frequently used to treat sinusitis and pneumonia. It is also useful in some types of skin infection (cellulitis) as well as in some types of bacterial diarrhea (*Salmonella, Shigella*).

*Preparation:* Suspension: 125, 250 mg/5ml. Capsule: 250, 500 mg

*Dosage:* INFANTS: 125 mg 4 times per day
TODDLERS: 125–250 mg 4 times per day
SCHOOL AGE: 250 mg 4 times per day
ADOLESCENTS: 250 mg 4 times per day

May be taken at any time but best absorption when taken on an empty stomach.

*Storage:*   Suspension requires refrigeration

*Side Effects:*   COMMON: Fine itchy, red rash—onset 2–3
days,* diarrhea,** yeast infection—
mouth or diaper area**
RARE: Hives***
SERIOUS ALLERGIC REACTION: Difficulty
breathing, low blood pressure***

*Comments:*   Ampicillin should not be given to a child with a
known allergy to penicillin.

## Aspirin

*Brand Names:*   Ascriptin, Bayer, Bufferin, and numerous
others

*Description and Uses:*   Aspirin is a salicyclate that is an
analgesic (antipain), an antipyretic (antifever), and anti-
inflammatory drug. The indications and mechanisms of action have been discussed in the sections on pain and fever.

*Preparations:*   There are *no* liquid aspirin preparations. Aspirin is available in combination with buffering chemicals or
antacids in buffered aspirin. However, there is no conclusive
evidence that buffered aspirin either protects the patient
from gastric irritation or increases the absorption or availability of aspirin to the body. It is also available in efferves-
cent tablets (Alka-Seltzer). Aspirin is both more rapidly absorbed and eliminated from the body in this form. Capsules
are used for patients with rheumatoid arthritis. Rectal suppositories are irritating. In general, we recommend only
plain aspirin for children. Most products are labeled in
grains (1 grain = 60 mg): baby aspirin: 1¼ grain or 80 mg;
most tablets: 5 grain or 300 mg; also available as 7½ grain
and 10 grain.

*Dosage:*   INFANTS: (less than six months consult a physician)
80 mg every 4 hours
TODDLERS: 160 mg every 4 hours

> School age: 240–400 mg every 4 hours
> Adolescents: 650 mg every 4 hours

If combined with acetaminophen, can be given at above dosage every 6 hours.

*Side Effects:*   Common: Gastric irritation***
>   Infrequent: Gastric ulcer,*** decreased blood component (platelet) count that may lead to increased bleeding tendency,*** wheezing,*** skin reactions***
>   Rare: Severe blistering,*** associated with Reye's syndrome***

*Comments:*   Ear-ringing is the sign of an overdose. When given with sulfonamides, aspirin may potentially increase their toxicity. *Aspirin is still a common cause of accidental overdose and death. Store away from children and in safety containers.* Flavored aspirin may encourage children to think of this potent medication as candy. Do *not* use for children who may have chicken pox or influenza.

## Baby Powders, Lotions, Creams, and Ointments

*Brand Names:*   *Powders:* Balmex Baby Powder, Diaperene Baby Powder, Formula Magic Lubricating Body Talc, Johnson and Johnson Baby Powder

*Lotions and creams*: Balmex emollient lotion, Keri cream, Keri lotion, Johnson & Johnson Baby cream

*Ointments:* A & D Ointment, Desitin ointment, Balmex ointment, Borofax ointment, Vaseline pure petroleum jelly, Zinc Oxide ointment

*Description and Uses:*   *Powders:* Powders act by reducing friction (lubricating) and absorbing moisture, both of which act to reduce irritation of the skin. They do not have healing powers and have not been conclusively shown to prevent or treat diaper rashes.

*Lotions and creams:* Cream and lotion act by lubricating and moisturizing the skin, and protecting the skin from irritations. It is thought, but not proven, that their actions help to prevent diaper rash.

*Ointments:* Ointments are felt to work by preventing evaporation of water from the skin, and protecting the skin from irritation. They also act as a barrier to keep irritants from contacting the skin. It is thought, but not proven, that this action helps to prevent diaper rash.

**Preparations:** *Baby powders:* These include one or more of the following ingredients: Talc, zinc oxide, zinc stearate, magnesium stearate, titanium oxide, gentonite, and calcium carbonate. Cornstarch can also be used as a baby powder.

*Lotions and creams:* These include one of the following ingredients: mineral oil, lanolin, talc, magnesium stearate, propylene paraben, and fragrances.

*Ointments:* These include one or more of the following ingredients: lanolin, petrolatum, cod liver oil, vitamins A and D, and talc.

**Dosage:** *Powder:* Apply to your hand first, and then to baby's bottom. Never dust directly onto the baby to avoid possible inhalation.

*Lotions and creams:* Apply a thin layer over the baby's bottom.

*Ointment:* Apply in a thin layer over the baby's bottom.

**Side Effects:** *Powder:* Talc can cause pneumonia if inhaled, and skin reactions if applied to bad wounds.

*Lotions and creams:* These preparations can cause a red rash secondary to an allergic reaction.

*Ointments:* The preparations can cause a red rash secondary to an allergic reaction.

**Comments:** Cornstarch is now marketed with fragrance at three times the price of cornstarch in the baking goods section. While it is as effective as the other powders, there is the slight risk of yeast thriving on the cornstarch.

## Beclomethasone

*Brand Names:* Beclovent, Vanceril Inhaler

*Description and Uses:* Beclomethansone is a drug of the steroid class, which when delivered to the respiratory tract as an inhalant is effective in reducing asthma symptoms in patients. It is preferable to oral dosages of steroids because many of the adverse effects of oral steroids do not accompany inhaled beclomethasone. However, higher dosages can cause suppression of the adrenal glands and other adverse consequences.

*Preparations:* Available as aerosols delivering 42 to 50 mcg/puff. (200 inhalations per container)

*Dosage:* INFANTS AND TODDLERS: Insufficient data to recommend dosages
SCHOOL AGE: 1 or 2 inhalations, 3 or 4 times daily
ADOLESCENTS: 2 to 4 inhalations, 3 or 4 times daily

*Side Effects:* COMMON: *Candida* infection***
INFREQUENT: Hoarseness,** dry mouth,** sore throat**

*Comments:* Special care must be taken if your child is on oral steroids and is being transferred to beclomethasone inhaler. This process usually takes several months. If your child develops a *Candida* yeast infection, this can be treated with nystatin or miconazole. Your physician may also wish to reduce the beclomethasone dosage.

If also using a bronchodilator inhaler to help your child breathe better, use it first, then wait several minutes before using this medicine.

Gargling and rinsing the mouth after each dose may help prevent hoarseness and throat irritation.

Do *not* discard the mouthpiece as refill canisters are available but brand named products are *not* interchangeable.

## Benzoyl Peroxide

*Brand Names:*  Benoxyl 5, 10, Benzac 5, 10, 5 Benzagel, 10 Benzagel, Desquam–X 5, 10, Loroxside, Oxy 5, 10, Persabel, Persadox-HP, Topex, Vanoxide, Xerac BP 5, 10. Other preparations, including Clearasil, have benzoyl peroxide in combination with other preparations.

*Description and Uses:*  This preparation is the initial drug of choice for management of most cases of mild to moderate acne. It is of proved efficacy and acts in several ways including antibacterial action against the bacterium responsible for acne (*Proprionibacterium acnes*). It is expected to cause mild irritation of the skin.

*Dosage:*  Begin applications initially at night. Leave preparation on for only 30 minutes, then wash with gentle soap. Advance until overnight application does not cause irritation. Avoid contact with eyes. Begin with 5% lotion or cream. If no effect is seen after daily preparations for 6 weeks, advance to 10% cream or lotion. If after 6 weeks of 10% cream or lotion applied all night there is no improvement, a gel may be recommended by your physician. Lotions and creams do not require a prescription.

*Side Effects:*  A mild irritation is expected. Up to 3% of people are sensitive (allergic) to benzoyl peroxide and will be unable to tolerate its use.

*Comments:*  Benzoyl peroxide may be used in combination with other acne therapy, including tretinoin. You may experience warmth after application. Avoid sensitive skin areas (eyelids, mouth). Allergy to hair bleach is an indicator of increased risk of allergy to benzoyl peroxide. Benzoyl peroxide may bleach hair or clothing.

## Brompheniramine

*Brand Names:* Dimetane, Symptom 3

*Description and Uses:* Brompheniramine is an antihistamine effective in the treatment of hay fever (seasonal allergic rhinitis). Of children with this condition, 75–90% will receive some symptomatic relief from this medication. Brompheniramine is also effective in the treatment of allergic "stuffy nose" (nonseasonal allergic rhinitis), but has not been proved effective in the treatment of the common cold. It has not been shown more or less effective than other antihistamines in the treatment of these conditions. It may be less effective than other types of antihistamines in the treatment of hives, but has been used in the treatment of other itchy skin disorders. It is a member of a class of antihistamines (alkylamines) that has the lowest incidence of associated drowsiness. This makes it a useful antihistamine for daytime use.

*Preparations:* Tablets: 4 mg; time-released, 8, 12 mg. Elixir: 2 mg/5 ml

*Dosage:* Regular tablets:
INFANTS: 0.5–1.0 mg every 6 hours
TODDLERS: 1.0 mg every 6 hours
SCHOOL AGE: 1.0–2.0 mg every 6 hours
ADOLESCENTS: 2.0–4.0 mg every 6 hours

Time-released tablets:
SCHOOL AGE: 8 mg every 12 hours
ADOLESCENTS: 8–12 mg every 8–12 hours

*Storage:* May be stored without refrigeration

*Side Effects:* COMMON: Drowsiness,* inability to concentrate*
INFREQUENT: Increased activity,* insomnia,* dizziness,*** nausea and vomiting,*** palpitations (heart skipping a beat, beating fast or irregularly)***

Rare: Frequent urination,** decreased production of blood products (look for easy bruising, frequent or serious infections),*** confusion,*** headaches,*** chills***

*Comments:* Because of the frequent behaviorial disturbances associated with the administration of antihistamines, care should be taken in giving this medication to children before school, skateboarding, rollerskating, bicycle riding, or operation of a potentially dangerous tool or toy. May take with food to decrease stomach upset. Do not chew, crush, or break time-released forms.

## Calamine Lotion

*Description and Uses:* Calamine lotion is one of several lotions used to relieve itching and to soothe skin that is not in a severe weeping state. Zinc oxide when combined with ferric oxide produces a pink mixture, calamine. Zinc oxide is also found by itself in many lotions. The lotions act principally by a cooling effect. They may also decrease the transmission of itch impulses coming from the nerves near the skin. Ingredients in various lotions include water, zinc oxide, talc, glycerin, and calamine. Some lotions may also contain agents with additional cooling or anti-itch properties including menthol, phenol, and camphor. The above chemicals are also available in ointments such as Desitin.

*Preparation:* Available as lotions in which ingredients must be mixed by shaking.

*Dosage:* Apply to skin surface. Do not use if skin has severe oozing. Do not use phenol on infants or young children.

*Side Effects:* Lotions with phenol should be applied only in small areas. Phenol can produce liver damage in infants. In high concentrations phenol may produce tumors. Talc may cause severe reactions on damaged skin.

*Comments:* Do not use lotions with antihistamines included, for they can irritate the skin.

## Cefaclor

*Brand Name:* Ceclor

*Description and Uses:* Cefaclor is a member of a group of antibiotics known as cephalosporins. It is effective against a wide variety of bacteria commonly responsible for infections in children. It is probably used most often in treating ear infections in children. Because it is effective against *Hemophilus influenzae* infections it may be used as a first-line drug in areas where there are many *Hemophilus* strains resistant to ampicillin. However, many other antibiotics are less costly. Although there is cross reactivity with penicillins, cephalosporins are regarded as alternatives for patients experiencing intolerance to the penicillins because of abdominal discomfort. Cefaclor kills streptococcal bacteria in pharyngitis, but its efficacy in preventing rheumatic fever has not been established.

*Preparations:* Concentrations: 125, 250 mg/5 ml. Capsules: 250, 500 mg

*Dosage:*   INFANTS: 100 mg 3 times a day
TODDLERS: 200 mg 3 times a day
SCHOOL AGE: 250 mg 3 times a day
ADOLESCENTS: 300 mg 3 times a day
May be taken with meals.

*Storage:* Suspension requires refrigeration. Suspension should be discarded after 14 days.

*Side Effects:*   INFREQUENT: Diarrhea,** nausea,** vomiting,** skin rash**
RARE: *Candida* vaginal infection,** diaper rash,** hives***

*Comments:* Children known to be allergic to other cephalosporins should not take this drug. Many children allergic to penicillin may be allergic to cefaclor.

For most infections cefaclor is not the first drug of choice; although it is as effective against ear and skin infections as more commonly used drugs, it is more expensive. Often when it is highly likely that two very different classes of bacterial organisms, such as *Hemophilus* and *Staphylococcus*, are present, either cefaclor may be used alone or two antibiotics like cloxacillin and ampicillin may be combined. The advantage of cefaclor is that as a single drug it is more expensive than either single alone, but cheaper than two. The disadvantage is that it does not offer the level of protection against more serious complications such as meningitis.

In certain situations when several bacteria are possible, your physician may use cefaclor alone, rather than combine two other drugs.

## Chicken Soup

*Brand Names:* _____ (fill in mother or grandmother's name), _____ (fill in mother-in-law's name)

*Description and Uses:* Chicken soup has been widely prescribed for a variety of illnesses, but mostly for colds and flu-like illnesses. Our mothers say it is unquestionably effective.

*Preparations:* Only "homemade" is effective.

*Dosage:* Give until child is full, then ask if they are sure they don't want a little more.

*Storage:* Should be refrigerated

*Side Effects:* Your mother or mother-in-law*

## Chloral Hydrate

*Brand Name:* Noctec

*Description and Uses:* Chloral hydrate is an effective sedative drug that may be useful in those situations in childhood when extreme circumstances (illness, injury, etc.) call for a medication to induce sleep. It has a rapid onset of action and is also eliminated from the body quickly. It loses its effectiveness after several weeks' use. It should not be used to regularly induce sleep.

*Preparations:*   Elixir: 500 mg/5 ml. Syrup: 250, 500 mg/5 ml. Capsules: 225, 250, 450, 500 mg. Suppositories: 460, 500 mg

*Dosage:*   INFANTS: 250 mg
TODDLERS: 500 mg
SCHOOL AGE: 1000 mg
ADOLESCENTS: 1000 mg

*Side Effects:*   INFREQUENT: Stomach irritation,\*\*\* hives\*\*\*
RARE: Excitement\*\*\*

*Comments:*   Chloral hydrate's unpleasant taste and odor can both be masked by chilling the liquid or by using other preparations. It may also be mixed with water, juice, or ginger ale.

### Chlorpheniramine Maleate

*Brand Names:*   Available in generic form, chlortrimeton, Histaspan, Teldrin

*Description and Uses:*   Chlorpheniramine is an antihistamine that is representative of a class of antihistamines called alkylamines. It is a common ingredient in cold medicines and is most commonly used in the treatment of upper-respiratory disorders. It is most effective in the management of hay fever (seasonal allergic rhinitis) with 70–95% of children receiving some symptomatic relief. Chlorpheniramine is also useful in the treatment of nonseasonal allergic rhinitis. Its effectiveness is unproved in the treatment of the common cold. Alkylamines will occasionally stimulate a child, causing increased activity, nervousness, tremors, and insomnia. Chlorpheniramine maleate can be used in the treatment of hives and itchy skin conditions. It is not as effective as other classes of antihistamines for these conditions, but it may be useful for daytime medication because of its low potential for sedation.

*Preparations:* Tablets: 4, 8, 12 mg; long-acting timed-release, 8, 12 mg. Timed-release capsules. Syrup: 2 mg/5 ml

*Dosage:*  INFANTS: See your physician
TODDLERS: 0.5–1.5 mg every 6 hours
SCHOOL AGE: 1.5–3.0 mg every 6 hours
ADOLESCENTS: 3.0–4.0 mg every 6 hours or 8–12 mg every 12 hours (timed-release form)

*Storage:*  May be stored without refrigeration

*Side Effects:*  COMMON: Drowsiness,* difficulty concentrating*
INFREQUENT: Increased activity,* insomnia,* nausea and vomiting,* dizziness,** tremors,** palpitations (heart skips a beat, or beats fast or irregularly)***
RARE: Frequent urination,** decreased production of blood products (look out for easy bruising, frequent or serious infections),*** confusion,*** headache,*** chills***

*Comments:*  Because of the infrequent behavior disturbances associated with giving antihistamines, care should be taken in giving this medication before school, when skateboarding, roller skating, riding a bicycle, or operating any potentially hazardous tool or toy. May be taken with food or milk to lessen stomach upset. Do not break, crush, or chew long-acting timed-release forms.


## Clotrimazole

*Brand Names:*  Gyne-Lotrimin, Lotrimin, Mycelex, Mycelex-G

*Description and Uses:* Clotrimazole is an antifungal agent effective in treating fungus infections of the skin (tinea corpus) in children and adolescents, candidal (yeast) vaginitis in postpubertal women, and candidal diaper rashes in infants. Clotrimazole has not been demonstrated to be more effective than any other topical antifungal drug, but it may be more effective than nystatin in the treatment of candidal vaginitis.

*Preparations:* Cream: 1% concentration. Solution: 1% concentration. Vaginal tablet: 100 mg

*Dosage: Fungus infection of the skin—Candida diaper rashes:* a thin layer of the cream or solution should be applied over the affected area twice a day. *Vaginitis:* one tablet or applicationful of cream is injected high in the vagina at night for 7 days. Or two tablets daily for three days. Use of sanitary napkin will prevent staining of clothing.

*Storage:* May be stored without refrigeration

*Side Effects:* INFREQUENT: Itching,** redness, burning, blistering of the skin***
RARE: Hives***

*Comments:* Use clotrimazole with caution around the eyes, for it can be irritating to the eye. Clotrimazole is not effective when used alone in fungus infections of the hair and nails.

## Cloxacillin and Dicloxacillin

*Brand Names:* Cloxapen, Dycill, Dynapen, Pathocil, Tegopen, Veracillin

*Description and Uses:* Cloxacillin and dicloxacillin are antibiotics that are related to penicillin and that are particularly effective in treating infections caused by *Staphylococcus* bacteria. In treating children they are generally used against skin infections including boils (furuncles), pustular diaper rash (rash with whiteheads), impetigo characterized by large pus-filled blisters and deep skin infections (abscesses). They are frequently used to treat infected lymph glands. They are also occasionally used when ear infections are suspected to be caused by *Staphylococcus*. Staphylococcus pneumonia is a severe problem that will require hospitalization.

| *Preparations:* | | *Dicloxacillin* | *Cloxacillin* |
|---|---|---|---|
| | Capsules: | 125, 250 mg, and 500 mg | 250, 500 mg |
| | Suspension: | 62.5 mg/5 ml | 125 mg/5 ml |

| *Dosage:* | | *Dicloxacillin* | *Cloxacillin* |
|---|---|---|---|
| | INFANTS: | 45 mg | 90 mg |
| | TODDLERS: | 62.5 mg | 125 mg |
| | SCHOOL AGE: | 250 mg | 250 mg |
| | ADOLESCENTS: | 250 mg | 250 mg |

*Storage:*  Suspension requires refrigeration

*Side Effects:*  INFREQUENT: Diarrhea,** nausea,** hives***
RARE: Serious allergic reaction characterized by difficulty breathing, dizziness, pallor***

*Comments:*  Dicloxacillin and cloxacillin are comparable in their therapeutic effectiveness in treating infections. These medicines should not be given to children with known penicillin allergy. Best absorption when taken 1 hour before or 2 hours after meals.


## Codeine

*Brand Names:*  Available generically in tablets or in combination products. Actified-C Expectorant, Ambenyl Expectorant, Calcidrine, Cerose, Colrex Compound, Dimetane Expectorant—DC, Histadyl E.C., Isoclor Expectorant, Novahistine Expectorant, Novahistine DH, Nucofed, Pediacof, Phenergan Expectorant with codeine, Ptenergan VC with codeine, Robitussin A–C, Robitussin DAL, Terpin Hydrate and Codeine Elixir, Triaminic Expectorant with Codeine, Tussan–2, Tussan SF, Tussi-organidin Expectorant

*Description and Uses:* Codeine is considered by many experts the most effective anticough drug available. Although codeine is a narcotic, the risk of drug dependency or addiction is considerably less than with morphine and heroin. In doses prescribed to suppress cough, the chance of developing drug addiction are astonishingly small.

*Preparations:* Tablets: 15, 30, 60 mg. Codeine in combination with other medicines vary in amounts from 10 mg to 20 mg for capsules and tablets, and from 5 mg to 20 mg per 5 ml of liquid.

*Dosage:* INFANTS: See your physician
TODDLERS: 2.5–5.0 mg every 6 hours
SCHOOL AGE: 5.0–10 mg every 6 hours
ADOLESCENTS: 10–20 mg every 6 hours

*Storage:* See labels on individual cough preparations.

*Side Effects:* COMMON: Drowsiness,* constipation,* nausea and vomiting**
RARE: Itching,** excessive salivating**

*Comments:* Be careful when taking codeine preparations with other medicines that can cause sedation such as antihistamines, for the effects can be additive. If possible, try not to give codeine preparations to your child during the day, for this may interfere with play or school performance.

## Cromolyn

*Brand Name:* Intal

*Description and Uses:* Cromolyn is unique among drugs used for asthma. It *cannot relieve an attack* but it is used to prevent attacks. It acts by preventing the release of chemicals known to constrict airways. Cromolyn is used in two types of situations: (1) to prevent the intermittent attacks of asthma it is inhaled four times daily; (2) to prevent the wheezing that accompanies exercise in some asthmatics it is administered shortly before exercise. Cromolyn is both quite safe and effective. It has enabled some children to discontinue steroids needed to control severe asthma. In older children, it should always be tried before a child is placed on chronic steroids for asthma control.

*Preparation:* Available as a 20 mg capsule with cromolyn powder that must be used with a special oral turbo-inhaler known as a Spinhaler®. The capsule is punctured inside the Spinhaler® and a small propeller is driven by the force of an inhalation.

*Dosage:* Children old enough to use the inhaler (usually 5 years old or more) may benefit from cromolyn. Several inhalations will be necessary to utilize all the powder in the capsule. Your child's neck should be extended with gaze upward during inhalation. Exhalations should *not* be made through the Spinhaler®. Initial dosage calls for 4 capsules daily. This can later be reduced to the lowest amount that will prevent symptoms. If your child experiences coughing associated with cromolyn inhalation, your physician may recommend use of a metaproterenol or albuterol inhalant immediately (5 to 15 minutes) prior to cromolyn.

*Side Effects:* INFREQUENT: Throat irritation,* cough,* hoarseness*

RARE: Hives,*** muscle aches,*** diarrhea,*** pneumonia***

*Comments:* Do not swallow capsules. Gargling and rinsing the mouth after each dose may help prevent throat irritation, dryness, and hoarseness.

### Crotamiton

*Brand Name:* Eurax

*Description and Uses:* Crotamiton is an effective drug in the treatment of scabies infestations, as well as being an effective anti-itch agent. It has not been demonstrated to be more or less effective than other antiscabies medicines, but because of its relatively low incidence of serious side effects it has become the drug of choice for many physicians.

*Preparations:*  Cream: 10% concentration
Lotion: 10%

*Dosage:*  The preparation should be massaged into the skin of the whole body from the chin down. Avoid contact with eyes, mouth, anus, and the opening of the urethra (the tube through which urine flows from the bladder to the outside). Do not wash off the medicine. Reapply the crotamiton in 24 hours, and do not wash off until 48 hours following the last application. It may be necessary to repeat the treatment in one week. Clothing and bed linen should be changed the next morning.

*Storage:*  May be stored at room temperature

*Side Effects:*  INFREQUENT: Allergic or contact inflammation of the skin***

*Comments:*  Crotamiton is irritating to red, raw, peeling skin.

### Cyproheptadine

*Brand Name:*  Periactin

*Description and Uses:*  This drug is an antihistamine used principally for itchiness. It is useful in hives produced from exposure to cold.

*Preparations:*  Tablets: 4 mg. Syrup: 2 mg/5 ml

*Dosage:*  INFANTS: 1 mg 2 times a day
TODDLERS: 2 mg 2 to 3 times daily
SCHOOL AGE: 4 mg 2 to 3 times daily
ADOLESCENTS: 4–6 mg

*Side Effects:*  COMMON: Drowsiness*
INFREQUENT: Increased weight gain (has been used as an appetite stimulant)*

## Dextroamphetamine

*Brand Name:* Dexedrine

*Description and Uses:* Dextroamphetamine belongs to a class of drugs known as amphetamines, which affect both the cardiovascular and central nervous system. Dextroamphetamine is used in children to control attention-deficit disorders (hyperkinetic syndrome). It has been shown to decrease hyperactive behavior but is to be used only in conjunction with a full behavior management program. Learning may not improve despite reduction in hyperactivity and increase in attention span. Because of its numerous side effects, as well as potential for abuse, it is usually not the initial drug employed, but is often used after a trial of methylphenidate. It appears to be somewhat better than pemoline.

*Preparations:* Capsules: 10, 15 mg; timed-release, 15 mg
Tablets: 5 mg, 10 mg. Elixir: 5 mg/5 ml

*Dosage:* SCHOOL AGE AND ADOLESCENTS: 5 mg once or twice daily. May be increased to 5-mg weekly increments. Maximum 40 mg

*Side Effects:* COMMON: Nervousness,** insomnia,** dry mouth,** nausea,** constipation,** decreased appetite,** weight loss,** growth retardation,** tremors,*** increased heart rate and palpitations,*** dizziness ***
INFREQUENT: Diarrhea**
RARE: Psychosis,*** involuntary movements,*** depression***

*Comments:* Dextroamphetamine can increase the blood level of imipramine.


## Dextromethorphan Hydrobromide

*Brand Names:* Available generically as a powder. It is found in combination with other medicines in Cerose Compound, Cheracol D Cough Syrup, Dimacol, Dorcol Pediatric

Cough Syrup, Novahistine DMX, Phenergan Pediatric Expectorant, Robitussin CF, Robitussin DM, Rondec–DM, Triaminicol Cough Syrup, Trind DM, Tussagesic, Tuss 1–Organidin DM

*Description and Uses:* Dextromethorphan hydrobromide is an effective nonnarcotic cough suppressant. It acts on the cough center in the brain by suppressing the incoming "tickle" or stimulus.

*Preparations:* Common cough preparations contain anywhere from 3.3 mg to 15 mg/5 cc of dextromethorphan hydrobromide. Be careful not to exceed the recommended dose of the combination medicine on the bottle or prescribed by your physician even though your child may not be receiving the recommended dose of dextromethorphan hydrobromide given here. This may occur because another medicine in the preparation limits the amount that can be given without any toxic effects.

*Dosage:*

| Every 6–8 hours | | Every 4 hours | |
|---|---|---|---|
| INFANTS: | 2.5–5.0 mg | INFANTS: | do not give every 4 hrs. |
| TODDLERS: | 5.0–10 mg | TODDLERS: | 2.5–5.0 mg |
| SCHOOL AGE: | 10–15 mg | SCHOOL AGE: | 5.0–10 mg |
| ADOLESCENTS: | 15–30 mg | ADOLESCENTS: | 10–20 mg |

*Storage:* May be stored without refrigeration

*Side Effects:* INFREQUENT: Drowsiness,* nausea,** dizziness**

### Diazepam

*Brand Name:* Valium

*Description and Uses:* This is one of the most extensively used drugs in its class (benzodiazepines) and in the United States. It is effective principally as an antianxiety drug for adults, but it may be used as a sedative for children in those unusual circumstances (severe illness or injury) when it may be desirable to induce sleep. As a class, benzodiazepines are effective and safer than nondiazepines commonly used as sedatives. Although another benzodiazepine has a shorter duration of time in the body (Oxazepam or Serax) data on its use in children are limited and it should not be used in children less than six years old.

*Preparations:* Tablets: 2, 5, 10 mg

*Dosage:*  SCHOOL AGE: 1 to 2 mg several hours before sleep
ADOLESCENTS: 1 to 5 mg several hours before sleep

*Side Effects:*  COMMON: Daytime sedation,* dizziness,*** headache,*** gait disturbance***
INFREQUENT: Constipation,** skin rash,*** fever,*** blurred vision,*** urinary incontinence,*** slurred speech,*** muscle tremor***
RARE: Aggressive behavior,*** blood disorders***

*Comments:*  *Do not use with any of the following:* Antihistamines, codeine, imipramine, or alcohol. May be taken with meals to decrease stomach upset.

## Dimetapp

*Combination Drug:* Brompheniramine, phenylephrine, phenylpropanolamine

*Description and Uses:*  Brompheniramine is an antihistamine; phenylephrine and phenylpropanolamine are adrenergic drugs in the sympathomimetic class. These drugs all have the individual ability to dry the nasal lining and may have additive effects when combined. They should not be used to counteract each other's side effects (drowsiness versus nervousness and insomnia).

*Preparations:* Elixir: bropheniramine 4 mg, phenylephrine 5 mg, phenylpropanolamine 5 mg/ 5 ml. Tablets: brompheniramine 12 mg, phenylephrine 15 mg, phenylpropanolamine 15 mg

*Dosage:* INFANTS: ½ teaspoon 3 times daily
TODDLERS: 1 teaspoon 3 to 4 times daily
SCHOOL AGE: 1–2 teaspoons 3 to 4 times daily
ADOLESCENTS: 2 teaspoonfuls 3 to 4 times daily or one tablet 2 times daily

*Side Effects:* See brompheniramine, phenylephrine, phenolpropanolamine

## Diphenhydramine Hydrochloride

*Brand Names:* Benadryl; Benylin syrup

*Description and Uses:* Diphenhydramine hydrochloride is an antihistamine that is most frequently used in the treatment of allergic reactions, hives, and itchy skin rashes. It is also effective in the treatment of hay fever (seasonal allergic rhinitis), allergic conjunctivitis, allergic stuffy nose (nonseasonal allergic rhinitis), but it is not routinely used for these conditions because of the increased incidence of drowsiness associated with this antihistamine. Diphenhydramine hydrochloride has not been shown to be effective in the treatment of the common cold.

Diphenhydramine hydrochloride is an effective cough suppressant, but in some comparative studies it is not as effective as codeine. It most likely acts on the cough center in the brain, and may also have a numbing effect on the back of the throat and airways, where the tickle of a cough originates.

*Preparations:* Capsules: 25 and 50 mg. Elixir: 12.5 mg/5 ml

*Dosage:*   Allergy:             Cough:

INFANTS: See your physician   INFANTS: Consult your
                                    physician

TODDLERS: 12.5–15.0 mg     TODDLERS: 3–6.25 mg every 4
    every 6 hours                hours

SCHOOL AGE: 12–50 mg      SCHOOL AGE: 6.25–12.5 mg
    every 6 hours              every 4 hours

ADOLESCENTS: 20–50 mg    ADOLESCENTS: 12.5–25 mg
    every 6 hours              every 4 hours

*Storage:* Diphenhydramine hydrochloride may be stored without refrigeration.

*Side Effects:* COMMON: Drowsiness,* inability to concentrate*

INFREQUENT: Increased activity,* insomnia,* dizziness,*** nausea and vomiting,*** palpitations (heart skipping a beat, or beating rapidly or irregularly)***

RARE: Decreased production of blood products (look for easy bruising or frequent or serious infections),*** headaches,*** chills,*** confusion,*** frequent urination***

*Comments:* Take with food to decrease stomach upset.

## Diphenoxylate Hydrochloride with Atropine

*Brand Names:* Colonil, Lomotil

*Description and Uses:* This drug has been shown to decrease the movement of material in the intestines and therefore to provide a decrease in the symptom of diarrhea. It is as effective as other agents such as opiates (codeine) and paregoric (a form of opium) but it does not have the same potential for abuse. To prevent potential abuse, atropine is added. Atropine produces dry mouth and flushing. Although effective, there are many side effects including fatal reactions. Infants and young children may encounter severe respiratory depression. In general, we feel that this agent has an extremely limited role and only then for older children or adolescents.

*Preparations:* Tablets: 2.5 mg diphenoxylate, 0.025 mg atropine. Liquid: 2.5 mg diphenoxylate, 0.025 mg atropine/ 5 cc

*Dosage:* Children over ten years: 2 mg every 5–6 hours

*Side Effects:* INFREQUENT: Dry mouth,* blurred vision,** intestinal blockage,*** rash,*** nausea,*** dizziness ***
RARE: Toxic colon distention,*** respiratory depression***

## Docusate

*Brand Names:* Colace (docusate sodium), Dialose (docusate potassium), Kasof, Surfak (docusate calcium)

*Description and Uses:* These laxatives are considered wetting agents and are useful in constipation. They soften stools. They may be useful in some situations where the first-line approach of using a bulk-forming agent, such as bran, has failed.

*Preparations:* Capsules: 50, 100, 250 mg. Drops: 10 mg/ml. Syrup: 20 mg/5 ml

*Dosage:* TODDLERS: 50 mg daily
SCHOOL AGE: 50–100 mg daily
ADOLESCENTS: 50–360 mg daily

Do not give for longer than one week. Do not use if child has abdominal pain.

*Side Effects:* INFREQUENT: Diarrhea***

*Comments:* Colace is sometimes recommended by physicians also for softening ear wax prior to removal. This is acceptable on a single occasion but should not be done routinely, for Colace may irritate the ear canal. Give with milk, juice, or infant formula to mask taste and maintain adequate fluid intake.

## Electrolyte and Fluid Replacements

*Brand Names:*  Lytren, Pedialyte

*Description and Uses:*  These liquids are used in mild cases of diarrhea to replace the loss of water and electrolytes in diarrhcal fluids. They should be used only for a day or two. They should not be used in severe vomiting or in severe dehydration. They also contain sugar in the form of dextrose but are inadequate nutritional sources.

*Preparations:*  Liquid in various sizes from 4 ounces to 32 ounces

*Dosage:*  As much as child will tolerate for 1–2 days. No more than 120 ml (4 oz.) per kg (2.2 lbs.)

*Side Effects:*  None

## Emetrol

*Ingredients:*  Levulose, dextrose, orthophosphoric acid

*Description and Uses:*  An over-the-counter preparation reported to be useful for vomiting. No studies exist demonstrating either superior safety or effectiveness over single-entity preparations. Not recommended.

*Comments:*  Emetrol is often recommended because it is not a phenothiazine antiemetic, which often has side effects that may obscure the true diagnosis of a child vomiting from a central nervous system disease. Although Emetrol is not responsible for this type of side effect, its efficacy is not clear. Vomiting can usually be alleviated by dietary restriction and usually ends on its own.

## Ephedrine Sulfate

*Brand Names:* Available generically or in combination with other drugs as Amsec, Bronkolixir, Bronkotabs, Isuprel Compound, Marax, Mudrane, Quadrinal, Quibron Plus, and Tedral

*Description and Uses:* Ephedrine sulfate is one of the older adrenergic broncholdilators that are not as effective or long-acting as the newer, more selective adrenergic drugs (metaproterenol, terbutaline). It also has numerous undesirable effects such as increased heart rate and nervous system stimulation. Because of undesirable effects ephedrine was often combined with sedative drugs to counteract these stimulant problems.

*Preparations:* Capsules: 25, 50 mg. Syrup; 11, 20 mg/5 ml

*Dosage:* INFANTS: ½ teaspoon every 6 hours of 11 mg/5 ml preparation
TODDLERS: 3/4 teaspoon every 6 hours of 11 mg/5 ml preparation
SCHOOL AGE: 1 teaspoon every 6 hours of 20 mg/5 ml preparation
ADOLESCENTS: 20–50 mg every 4 to 6 hours

*Side Effects:* COMMON: Nervousness,*** excitability,*** insomnia***
INFREQUENT: Palpitations,*** increased heart rate***

*Comments:* Ephedrine sulfate offers no advantages over newer adrenergic drugs and has far more frequent undesired effects. There is no sense in counteracting these effects with sedatives—other single adrenergic agents are always preferred to ephedrine sulfate and these combination drugs.

## Ephinephrine, Advenaline *(inhalant)*

*Brand Names:* Adrenalin Chloride, Medihaler-Epi, microNEFRIN, Vaponefrine

*Description and Uses:*   As an injection, epinephrine is a mainstay in treating asthma. It is an adrenergic drug that opens bronchi, constricts blood vessels, and relieves the swelling of the bronchi. However it has numerous effects on the heart. Although it is available without prescription in aerosolized form it is not the preferred drug for oral inhalation. In addition to cardiac effects it can irritate the sensitive bronchial linings.

*Preparation:*   Several forms of epinephrine are available in nonprescription metered-dose inhalers. We do not recommend their use.

*Dosage:*   We do not recommend use. If all other forms of asthma therapy have resulted in adverse reactions, an unlikely event, this may be acceptable therapy. Consult your physician for recommendations.

*Side Effects:*   INFREQUENT: Tolerance,** anxiety,*** palpitation,*** rapid heart rate,*** muscle tremor,*** headache***


## Erythromycin

*Brand Names:*   *Erythromycin:* E-Mycin, Ilotycin, Robimycin, RP-Mycin, *Erythromycin estolate,* Ilosone: *Erythromycin ethylsuccinate:* E.E.S., Pediamycin; *Erythromycin stearate:* Bristamycin, Erythrocin stearate, Erypar, Ethril, Pfizer-E, *Topicals:* A/T/S, Eryderm, Staticin

*Description and Uses:*   Erythromycin is one of the safest antibiotics available today, and it is used in a wide range of infections. It is an effective antibiotic in the treatment of skin infections (some *Staphylococcus* infections may be resistant to erythromycin). It is also used for treatment of strep throat for those children who are allergic to penicillin. It has been used effectively as an initial drug in treatment of pneumonias in school-age children. It has been combined with sulfa antibiotics to treat middle-ear infections and has been used to treat certain types of venereal disease in adolescents. It has also been used both orally and topically in the treatment of acne. There is little difference among the preparations except that the estolate version has been reported to cause a reversible hepatitis. This has been reported to occur primarily in adults.

*Preparations:*   *Erythromycin estolate:* Suspension: 125, 250 mg/5 ml, Tablets: 125, 250, 500 mg, Capsules: 125, 250 mg

*Erythromycin:* Tablets: 250, 500 mg. Enteric coated tablets: 250, 333 mg

*Erythromycin ethylsuccinate:* Suspension: 200, 400 mg/5 ml, Tablets: (chewable) 200 mg

*Erythromycin stearate:* tablets: 250, 500 mg

*Erythromycin topical:* 1.5%, 2% solution

*Dosage:*   *Infechant:*

INFANTS: 72.5 mg every six hours
TODDLERS: 125 mg every six hours
SCHOOL AGE: 250 mg every six hours
ADOLESCENTS: 250–500 mg every six hours

*Acne*: Apply twice a day

*Side Effects:*   COMMON (oral): Mild nausea,* stomach cramping,* diarrhea**
COMMON (topical): Redness,** dryness,** burning and itching**
INFREQUENT: Vomiting,** heartburn**
RARE: Skin rashes,** hepatitis (with estolate preparations)***

*Comments:*   When using topical erythromycin wash and dry areas to be treated before each use. Avoid application near eyes, nose, and mouth. Erythromycin estolate, ethylsuccinate, enteric coated may be taken with meals to decrease gastrointestinal upset. Erythromycin and erythromycin stearate should be taken 1 hour before or 2 hours after meals.

### Erythromycin/Sulfisoxazole

*Brand Name:*  Pediazole

*Description and Uses:*  Pediazole is a combination of two well known antibiotics that was designed to be an alternative drug for treatment of otitis media. It is used where there is allergy to amoxicillin/ampicillin or where there is suspected bacterial resistance. Because of the combined side effects of two drugs, it is not recommended as an initial drug for this condition. Some physicians also use this drug combination for initial treatment of non-viral pneumonia.

*Preparation:*  Suspension: 200 mg erythromycin/600 mg sulfisoxazole per 5 ml. Strawberry-banana flavor

*Dosage:*  INFANTS: ¼–½ Tsp every 6 hours
TODDLERS: ½–1 Tsp every 6 hours
SCHOOL AGE: 1–1½ Tsp every 6 hours
ADOLESCENTS: 2 Tsp every 6 hours

*Storage:*  Pediazole needs to be refrigerated.

*Side Effects:*  COMMON: Nausea,* vomiting,* heartburn*
INFREQUENT: Headache,** skin rash***
RARE: Yellowing of eyes and skin (hepatitis),*** fatigue, pallor (anemia),*** behavior disorders***

*Comments:*  This medicine may be taken with meals to minimize stomach irritation. If your child is taking theophylline for asthma, let your physician know. He may need to adjust the theophylline dosage to avoid possible toxicity.

### Ethosuximide

*Brand Name:*  Zarontin

*Description and Uses:*  Ethosuximide is the drug of choice for the treatment of petit mal seizure in children. It has also been used in the treatment of other unusual seizure disorders in children.

*Preparations:* Syrup: 250 mg/5 ml. Capsules: 250 mg (raspberry flavor)

*Dosage:* SCHOOL AGE: 250 mg daily
ADOLESCENTS: 500 mg daily

*Side Effects:* COMMON: Nausea,** vomiting,** loss of appetite**
INFREQUENT: Drowsiness,** headache,** euphoria,** skin rash,** change in behavior,** dizziness***
RARE: Decreased production of blood and platelets, frequent and easy bruising, fatigue, pallor***

*Comments:* May be taken with food or milk.


## Glycerine Suppository

**Brand Name:** Available generically

**Description and Uses:** Glycerine suppositories are a stimulant form of laxative that both softens hardened fecal matter and stimulates a reflex to promote defecation. It may be used in certain situations if the first-line bulk-forming agent, bran, or prune juice is ineffective. It also may be used regularly for children who soil their underpants as a means of re-establishing reflex bowel activity. The suppository usually works within 15–30 minutes.

*Preparations:* Suppositories: 1, 1.5, 3 gm

*Dosage:* TODDLERS: 1 gm suppository
SCHOOL AGE: 1.5 gm suppository
ADOLESCENTS: 3 gm suppository

Do not use longer than one week. Do not use if child has abdominal pain.

*Side Effects:* INFREQUENT (with chronic usage): Diarrhea,*** dependence***

## Griseofulvin

*Brand Names:* *Ultramicrocrystalline form:* Fulvicin P/G, Gris–PEG. *Microcrystalline form:* Fulvicin–V/F, Grifulvin V, Grisactin

*Description and Uses:* Griseofulvin is an antifungal agent related to penicillin that is active against most fungi affecting the skin, hair, and nails. It is not effective against *Candida* or yeast. Griseofulvin is taken orally, and absorbed by the body. This enables it to be active against fungi within the hair and nails that cannot be reached by topical antifungals. Because of this, it is the drug of choice for fungus infections in these areas.

*Preparations:* Griseofulvin is marketed in forms related to the size of the basic crystal: microcrystalline form, and ultramicrocrystalline form. Theoretically the smaller the crystal, the greater the level of the drug achieved in the blood that can be achieved at a given dose. Practically there have been no demonstrated differences in effectiveness between the two preparations in treating fungus infections. Tablets: microcrystalline, 125, 250, 500 mg; ultramicrocrystalline, 125, 250 mg. Suspension: 125 mg/15 ml

| *Dosage:* | Microcrystalline form | Ultramicrocrystalline form |
|---|---|---|
| INFANTS: | 60 mg/day | 30 mg/day |
| TODDLERS: | 100–150 mg/day | 50–75 mg/day |
| SCHOOL AGE: | 200–500 mg/day | 100–250 mg/day |
| ADOLESCENTS: | 500 mg–1.0 gm/day | 250–500 mg/day |

Griseofulvin may be given once a day, or in divided doses with meals but must be continued for from 4 weeks up to 6 months depending upon the site of infection.

*Side Effects:* COMMON: Headaches,** nausea,** vomiting,** diarrhea**

INFREQUENT: Increased sensitivity to sun and sunlamps,** dizziness,*** fever,*** inflammation of the nerve (evident as pain,

tingling, weakness of part of the body),\*\*\*
joint pain\*\*\*

RARE: Decreased production of blood products (white blood cells—evident as frequent or serious infections),\*\*\* fainting spells,\*\*\* blurry vision,\*\*\* inflammation of the liver (evident as fatigue, yellow jaundice)\*\*\*

*Comments:* Some physicians recommend routine analysis of blood when prescribing griseofulvin for long periods of time to detect possible side effects before they become a serious problem.

## Haloprogin

*Brand Name:* Halotex

*Description and Uses:* Haloprogin is an antifungal agent that is highly effective in the treatment of fungus infections of the skin. It may be more effective, with fewer relapses, than tolnaftate in the treatment of those infections.

*Preparations:* Cream: 1% concentration. Solution: 1% concentration

*Dosage:* Haloprogin cream or solution is applied liberally to the affected area twice a day. Most fungus infections of the skin are responsive in 2–3 weeks. Lesions between the fingers may need up to four weeks of treatment.

*Storage:* May be stored at room temperature

*Side Effects:* INFREQUENT: Local irritation,\*\*\* burning sensation,\*\*\* formation of blisters\*\*\*

*Comments:* Caution should be used when applying haloprogin around the eyes, for it can be extremely irritating to the eyes. Haloprogin is not effective when used alone in fungus infections of the hair or nails.

## Hydroxyzine

*Brand Names:* Atarax, Vistaril

*Description and Uses:* Hydroxyzine is an antihistamine that has a number of properties that make it useful for anxiety, vomiting, and itching caused by allergic skin conditions. It is most often used in children for this latter condition.

*Preparations:* Tablets and capsules: 10, 25, 50, 100 mg. Syrups: (Atarax) 10 mg/5 ml. Suspension: (Vistaril) 25 mg/5 ml

*Dosage:* INFANTS: 2.5 mg 4 times daily
TODDLERS: 5 mg 4 times daily
SCHOOL AGE: 10–15 mg 4 times daily
ADOLESCENTS: 15–25 mg 4 times daily

*Side Effects:* COMMON: Drowsiness*
INFREQUENT: Dry mouth*

*Comments:* May take with meals.


## Imipramine

*Brand Names:* Imarate, SK–Pramine, Tofranil, Tofranil–PM

*Description and Uses:* This tricyclic drug is used for the treatment of depression in adults but is primarily used for the management of bedwetting in children. The mechanism of action is unclear. Imipramine may alter the way the bladder sphincter muscle operates, or it may alter sleep patterns.

*Preparations:* Tablets: 10, 25, 50 mg. Capsules: 75, 100, 125, 150 mg

*Dosage:* SCHOOL-AGE AND ADOLESCENTS: 10 mg nightly for one week. If no decrease in bedwetting, can be increased 10 mg weekly up to the following maximum doses:
8-YEAR-OLDS: 50 mg

10-YEAR-OLDS: 60 mg
12-YEAR-OLDS: 70 mg
14-YEAR-OLDS: 75 mg

*Side Effects:*   COMMON: Drowsiness,** dry mouth,** nausea or vomiting,** constipation,** visual disturbances,** sleep difficulty,** behavior changes**

Withdrawal reactions after prolonged use include fatigue, headaches, and nausea

*Comments:*   Best given ½ hour before bedtime. May be taken with food or milk. A gradual decrease in dosage is less likely to lead to a relapse than sudden withdrawal.


## Ipecac

*Description and Uses:*   Ipecac acts on both the stomach and the vomiting center in the brain to induce vomiting. An adequate dose causes vomiting in 30 minutes in 90% of children. The vomiting comes more quickly if 4–6 ounces of water is given prior to or just after giving the ipecac. Most physicians recommend that parents have ipecac syrup in the house by the time their child reaches 1 year of age to treat accidental poisonings. When treating poisonings remember *first* to call your regional poison control center or your physician before administering ipecac. For some substances, such as furniture oil or gasoline, stimulating vomiting may be harmful.

*Preparations:*   15 ml and 30 ml containers (non-prescription), 120 ml containers (prescription)

*Dosage:*   INFANTS 9–12 MONTHS: 10 ml (two teaspoons)
CHILDREN 1–12 YEARS OF AGE: 15 ml (one tablespoon)
ADOLESCENTS: 20 ml

The dose may be repeated *once* if vomiting has not occurred in 30 minutes.

*Side Effects:*  RARE: Overdosage with ipecac may cause serious disturbances in the rhythm of the heart beat***

*Comments:*  Ipecac can always be safely taken for an overdose of a medicine.


## Iron (Ferrous Sulfate)

*Brand Names:*  Feosol, Fer-In-Sol, Fero-Gradumet, Mol-Iron

*Description and Uses:*  Ferrous sulfate is used to treat iron-deficiency anemia in children who lack sufficient iron in their diet or who have reasons for excess blood loss and therefore require extra iron. The most common reason for iron deficiency in children is the feeding of excess milk (which is a poor iron source) to an infant or a toddler.

*Preparations:*  5 mg of ferrous sulfate provides 1 mg of elemental iron. Capsules: 150 mg (30 mg elemental iron), 250, 390 mg. Tablets: 325 mg (65 mg elemental iron), 525 mg. Elixir: 220 mg (44 mg elemental iron)/5 ml, 245 mg/5ml. Syrup: 90 mg (18 mg elemental iron)/5 ml. Drops: 75 mg (15 mg elemental iron)/0.6 ml

**Note:** These are therapeutic, *not* preventive doses.

*Dosage:*  INFANTS: 125 mg (25 mg elemental iron) daily, divided into 3 or 4 doses, for 1–2 months
TODDLERS: 250 mg (50 mg elemental iron) daily, divided into 3 or 4 doses, for 1–2 months
SCHOOL AGE: 500 mg (100 mg elemental iron) daily, divided into 3 or 4 doses, for 1–2 months
ADOLESCENTS: 1200 mg (240 mg elemental iron) daily, divided into 3 or 4 doses, for 1–2 months

*Side Effects:*  COMMON: Black stools,* stomach irritation,** nausea,** diarrhea,** constipation**

*Comments:*  Care should be used in iron storage. As few as

6 adult tablets may be fatal to young children. Although ferrous sulfate is absorbed best between meals, intestinal side effects can be minimized by giving during or shortly after meals. Liquid iron preparations may be diluted in or taken with water or juice to prevent staining of teeth and to mask taste.

## Isoniazid

*Brand Names:*   INH, Nydrazid

*Description and Uses:*   Isoniazid is an antibiotic used in the treatment and prevention of active tuberculosis. One of the most effective drugs used to treat tuberculosis, it is almost always used with another antituberculosis drug in order to prevent the emergence of tuberculosis bacteria resistant to isoniazid. Isoniazid is most commonly used in pediatrics to prevent the development of symptomatic tuberculosis after your child has been exposed to tuberculosis. If your child has a positive tuberculosis skin test, this indicates that he or she has been exposed to tuberculosis and that most often his or her body has already suppressed the infection. Treatment with isoniazid at this time for one year will greatly reduce the likelihood of active tuberculosis developing in your child.

*Preparations:*   Suspension: 50 mg/15 ml. Tablets: 100, 300 mg

*Dosage:*   INFANTS: 60 mg, once a day
TODDLERS: 100–150 mg, once a day
SCHOOL AGE: 200 mg, once a day
ADOLESCENTS: 300 mg, once a day

*Side Effects:*   COMMON: Inflammation of the liver (this usually causes no symptoms and is not harmful to children),** inflammation of the nerves (evident as pain, weakness, tingling),*** bizarre behavior***
INFREQUENT: Joint pain, with and without swelling***

> RARE: Damage to the optic nerve (evident as disturbance in vision—in particular color vision),\*\*\* convulsions\*\*\*

*Comments:*  Your doctor may want your child to take pyridoxine ($B_6$) with your INH to prevent or lessen some of the side effects.

## Isoproterenol

*Brand Names:*  Isuprel Mistometer, Medihaler-Iso, Norisodrine Sulfate

*Description and Uses:*  This adrenergic drug has been used for years as an effective treatment and preventive for bronchoconstriction in asthma. However, it is neither as selective nor as long-acting as the newer drugs metaproterenol sulfate and terbutaline. It has been widely abused in the past; tolerance often develops and problems have occurred from cardiac irregularities. Sudden deaths from overuse were in part due to a propellant no longer in use.

*Preparations:*  Solutions: 1:100 to 1:400. Powders: 10 mg and 25 mg cartridge for inhalation.

*Dosage:*  Isoproterenol is delivered in preset doses from hand-held nebulizers. It also is administered from mechanical ventilators and nebulizers. Hand-held nebulizer usage requires the ability to take a prolonged inhalation through the mouth. Following inhalation your child should hold his or her breath for several seconds. These tasks are suitable only for older children.

> SCHOOL AGE AND ADOLESCENTS: The least number of inhalations of the 1:200 solution. No more than 10 daily. Adult supervision required.

*Side Effects:*  COMMON: Dry mouth,\*\* nervousness,\*\* insomnia\*\*

> INFREQUENT: Sweating,\*\* palpitations,\*\*\*

rapid heart rate,\*\*\* irregular heart beat,\*\*\* dizziness,\*\*\* nausea,\*\*\* vomiting,\*\*\* stomach pain,\*\*\* increased asthma symptoms \*\*\*

*Comments:* Isoproterenol inhalants are accompanied by frequent unwanted effects. They also promote psychological dependence. Newer, more selective inhalants are preferable for attempted immediate relief from asthma attacks.

## Kaolin/Pectin

*Brand Name:* Kaopectate

*Description and Uses:* Kaolin is a form of clay, and pectin is a natural binding ingredient found in food such as apples. These products are often combined to control diarrhea. There is no evidence that the amount of fluid loss is decreased, but stool consistency may change from a liquid to a semisoft consistency. If this feature is important to you, kaolin/pectin mixtures can be used with the knowledge that they are quite safe.

*Preparation:* Kaopectate: 900 mg Kaolin and 20 pectin/5 ml. Kaopectate concentrate: 1350 mg Kaolin and 30 mg pectin/5 ml

*Dosage:* Do not use longer than 2 days. Do not use under the age of three years.
THREE TO SIX YEARS: 15 ml concentrate after each loose bowel movement
SCHOOL AGE: 30 ml concentrate
ADOLESCENTS: 45 ml concentrate

*Side Effects:* INFREQUENT: Constipation,\*\* impaction in infants\*\*\*

*Comments:* Kaolin or pectin may interfere with the absorption of other medications and should not be administered simultaneously with other therapy.

**Lindane** *(Gamma Benzene Hexachloride)*

*Brand Names:* GBH, Kwell

*Description and Uses:* Lindane is an effective drug against both scabies and all types of lice. It has not been documented to be more or less effective than other commonly used drugs against scabies and lice. It has, however, been shown that lindane can be absorbed through the skin. This absorption can be excessive if the lindane is applied over inflamed or denuded areas or if it is applied incorrectly or excessively. If this happens, convulsions and damage to the nervous system can occur. On the other hand, there has been widespread use of lindane for delousing in World War II, and during times of disaster, with little or no serious side effects reported.

*Preparations:* Cream, lotion, shampoo: 1% concentration. Powder: 6% concentration

*Dosage:* Because of the potential for toxic absorption of lindane we do not recommend it be used in children under the age of two years. *Scabies:* Following a soap-and-water bath, the skin should be thoroughly dried. Then apply the lotion or the cream in a thin layer to all parts of the body except the face. The lotion should be washed off after 6 to 8 hours. Retreatment may be necessary. *Head lice:* One ounce or less of the shampoo should be applied and worked into a lather, and the scalp shampooed for 5 minutes, then rinsed and dried. Treatment may need be repeated in one week if new eggs are seen, but not more than twice. *Pubic lice:* Following a soap-and-water bath, a thin layer of lotion should be applied to the pubic region including the area around the anus. In hairy individuals, the thighs, chest, and underarms should also be treated. The lotion should be washed off after 6 to 8 hours. A second application may be necessary in one week, if new eggs are seen. This medicine should not be applied more than twice. The shampoo is not as effective as the lotion for pubic lice.

*Side Effects:* INFREQUENT: Inflammation and redness of

skin with frequent and liberal applications***
RARE: Convulsions and damage to the central nervous system***—see section on description and use

## Mebendazole

*Brand Name:* Vermox

*Description and Uses:* Mebendazole is an antibiotic that is effective against a number of worms that infect children. It is one of the drugs of choice (along with pyrantel pamoate) in the treatment of pinworm. It is the drug of choice in the treatment of hookworm and whipworm.

*Preparation:* Tablets (chewable): 100 mg

*Dosage:* *Pinworm:* 100 mg for one dose for all children and adolescents. *Hookworm, whipworm:* 100 mg twice a day for 3 days for all children and adolescents

*Side Effects:* INFREQUENT: Abdominal pain,** diarrhea**

*Comments:* The effects of mebendazole in children under two years old has not been well studied. Consult your physician as to the risks and benefits of using it in a child of this age. Tablets may be crushed and mixed and given with food.

## Metaproterenol Sulfate

*Brand Names:* Alupent, Metaprel

*Description and Uses:* Metaproterenol is an effective bronchodilator that is a member of a class of drugs known as adrenergic drugs. Older adrenergic drugs such as ephedrine, isoproterenol, and isoetharine stimulate the heart and nervous system. Metaproterenol is more specific in its ability to selectively cause the bronchodilation desired for relief of asthma without incurring cardiac and nervous system stimulation. It is available as either an oral inhalant for immediate relief, or as a preventive as an oral tablet or syrup. Because of its greater selectivity and longer duration of action it is the first drug of choice as an inhalant and has largely replaced isopreterenol.

*Preparations:*  Micronized powder in a metered-dose inhaler. Syrup: 10 mg/5 ml. Tablets: 10, 20 mg

*Dosage:*  INFANTS AND TODDLERS: Limited information; consult your physician
SCHOOL AGE: 10 mg 3 to 4 times a day
ADOLESCENTS: 20 mg 4 times a day

*Side Effects:*  COMMON: Bad taste in mouth,** muscle tremor***
INFREQUENT: Drying of throat,* dizziness,** nausea,** vomiting,** nervousness,** rapid heart rate,*** palpitations***

*Comments:*  Metaproterenol is used as the first drug for treating chronic asthma in England. Recent studies suggest that because of its safety and efficacy it may take over the number one spot in this country from the current leader, theophylline. Save your applicator when using the inhalant. Refill units are available.

## Methylphenidate

*Brand Name:*  Ritalin

*Description and Uses:*  This drug is a central nervous system stimulant that is principally used as part of the management of children with attention deficit disorders (hyperkinetic syndrome). Although methylphenidate may increase attention span and decrease hyperactive behavior, it is still unclear whether learning will be improved. Ritalin is currently a first-line drug for attention deficits, for it seems to be more effective than pemoline (Cylert) and have fewer side effects and potential for abuse than dextroamphetamine (Dexedrine).

*Preparations:* Tablets: 5, 10, 20 mg

*Dosage:* SCHOOL AGE: 5 mg twice daily. May be increased to 10 mg twice daily. Maximum daily dose 40 mg
ADOLESCENTS: 10 mg twice daily. May be increased to 20 mg twice daily. Maximum daily dose 60 mg

*Side Effects:* COMMON: Weight loss,** growth retardation,** nervousness,** decreased appetite,** sleep disturbance***
INFREQUENT: Dizziness,** abdominal pain,** nausea,** increased heart rate or palpitations,*** skin rash***
RARE: Psychosis***

*Comments:* If despite adequate dosing (usually 0.5 mg/kg up to 2 mg/kg of your child's weight) there is no improvement in a month, the drug should probably be discontinued. Methylphenidate increases the toxicity of phenytoin and primidone and elevates the blood level of imipramine.


## Metronidazole

*Brand Name:* Flagyl

*Description and Uses:* Metronidazole is an antibiotic that is effective against Entamoeba and giardia infections in children. It is one of the drugs of choice (along with quinacrine) in the treatment of giardia, and one of the drugs of choice in amoeba infections of the gut and other organs. Metronidazole is also effective in a one-dose regimen in the treatment of *Trichomonas* vaginitis (vaginal discharge from trichomonad infection).

*Preparation:*   Tablets: 250 mg

*Dosage:*   *Amebiasis:*
INFANTS: 75–100 mg 3 times a day
TODDLERS: 100–250 mg 3 times a day
SCHOOL AGE: 250–500 mg 3 times a day
ADOLESCENTS: 500–750 mg 3 times a day
*Giardiasis:*
INFANTS: 10–15 mg 3 times a day
TODDLERS: 15–30 mg 3 times a day
SCHOOL AGE: 50–100 mg 3 times a day
ADOLESCENTS: 100–250 mg 3 times a day

*Storage:*   May be stored without refrigeration

*Side Effects:*   INFREQUENT: Nausea,** diarrhea,** unpleasant taste in mouth,** abdominal pain***
RARE: Furry tongue,** sores in mouth,*** dizziness,*** headache,*** hives,*** burning on urination,*** darkening of the urine,*** decreased production of white blood cells (look for frequent or serious infections)***

*Comments:*   Metronidazole has been found to cause cancer in mice and rats, but not in other animals. Most importantly, it has not been shown to cause cancer in man. Although these findings are of some concern, there is widespread belief that for the conditions described here metronidazole is the most effective and least toxic drug available. May be taken with meals to decrease stomach upset.


## Miconazole

*Brand Names:*   Micatin, Monistat-Derm (topical), Monistat 7 (intravaginal)

*Description and Uses:*   Miconazole is an antifungus preparation that is highly effective against fungus infections of the skin, fungus-caused (yeast, *Monilia*) diaper rashes, and in postpubertal women yeast-caused vaginitis. It is probably the drug of choice for yeast vaginitis, and a first-line drug for diaper rashes and fungus infections of the skin.

*Preparations:* Cream: 2% concentration. Lotion: 2% concentration

*Dosage:* *Fungus infections of the skin and diaper rash:* A thin layer of the cream (lotion may be used in hairy areas). Apply to affected skin in the morning and evening until the infection disappears. (If no improvement in 4 weeks, consider another diagnosis.)

*Yeast (Monilia) vaginitis:* One applicationful of cream injected high in the vagina at night for seven days. Use of a sanitary napkin will prevent staining of clothing.

*Storage:* May be stored without refrigeration

*Side Effects:* INFREQUENT: Irritation and burning***

*Comments:* Use miconazole cautiously around the eyes, for it may cause irritation. Miconazole is not effective alone in the treatment of fungus infections of the hair and nails.

### Neosporin Ointment

*Description and Uses:* This ointment is a combination of three antibiotics, bactitracin, polymyxin B, and neomycin, that are poorly absorbed and that are intended to treat superficial infections of the skin, e.g., superficial boils and impetigo. It is not effective in deep infections of the skin, e.g., cellulitis, deep-seated boils, or extreme impetigo. In general this ointment is not as effective as oral preparations of antibiotics in the treatment of skin infections. If Neosporin is used to treat skin infections, any crusting of the sore must be removed before application of the ointment. The antibiotic neomycin may also cause an allergic skin reaction.

*Dosage:* The ointment should be applied in a thin layer 3–4 times per day

*Side Effects:* INFREQUENT: Allergic contact dermatitis***

## Nitrofurantoin

*Brand Names:* Cyantin, Furadantin, Macrodantin, and others

*Description and Uses:* Nitrofurantoin is an antibiotic that is used almost exclusively for the treatment and prevention of urinary tract infections. Nitrofurantoin has been supplanted by newer antibiotics such as trimethoprim/sulfamethoxazole for these purposes and is rarely the first drug of choice.

*Preparations:* Suspension: 25 mg/15 ml. Tablets, capsules: 25, 50, 100 mg

*Dosage:*  INFANTS: 10 mg every 4 times a day
TODDLERS: 15–25 mg 4 times a day
SCHOOL AGE: 25–50 mg 4 times a day
ADOLESCENTS: 50–100 mg 4 times a day

*Side Effects:* COMMON: Nausea,** vomiting,** diarrhea,** fever**
INFREQUENT: Skin rash,*** hives,*** headache,*** drowsiness,*** dizziness,*** numbness, tingling, or burning of face***
RARE: Inflammation of the lung (evident as trouble breathing),*** decreased production of blood products (evident as fatigue, serious infection, unusual breathing),*** inflammation of the liver (evident as fatigue and yellow jaundice)

*Comments:* The macrocrystals (macrodantin) are less likely to cause the common side effects. Should be taken with food or milk to decrease stomach upset.

## Novahistine

*Combination Drug:* Chlorpheniramine (tablet and elixir),

phenylephrine (tablet), phenylpropanolamine (elixir)

*Description and Uses:* This combination drug contains ingredients effective in drying the nasal mucosa. Although it is of use in the symptom relief of colds, there is no known evidence that this drug is effective in preventing or treating ear infections.

*Preparations:* Elixir: 18.5 mg phenylpropanolamine, 2 mg chlorpheniramine. Tablet: 20 mg phenylephrine, 4 mg chlorpheniramine

*Dosage:*  INFANTS: ½ teaspoon 3 or 4 times daily
TODDLERS: 1 teaspoon 3 or 4 times daily
SCHOOL AGE: 1–2 teaspoons 3 or 4 times daily
ADOLESCENTS: 2–3 teaspoons or 1 tablet 3 or 4 times daily

*Side Effects:* *See* chlorpheniramine, phenylephrine, phenylpropanolamine

## Nystatin

*Brand Names:* Mycostatin, Nilstat, O-V Statin Candex

*Description and Uses:* Nystatin is an antibiotic that is effective against a variety of fungi, but it is used almost exclusively for the treatment of *Candida* (yeast) infections. For infants, it is used to treat *Candida* diaper rashes, and in adolescents it is effective against *Candida* vaginitis. It is highly effective in both these conditions, but it may be less effective than miconazole or clotrimazole in the treatment of vaginitis.

*Preparations:* Cream: 100,000 units/gram. Lotion, 100,000 units/milliliter. Powder, 100,000 units/gram. Ointment: 100,000 units/gram. Suspension: 100,000 units

*Dosage: Diaper rash:* Cream or lotion is applied over the affected area twice a day in a thin layer. For wet, moist skin, the powder is often preferred and is prescribed two or three times a day. One to two ml of oral suspension may be given four times daily for diaper rash. *Vaginitis:* One to two tablets or applicationful high in the vagina for 2 weeks

*Storage:* May be stored without refrigeration

*Side Effects:* INFREQUENT: May cause irritation of the skin,** diarrhea,** nausea,** vomiting** (with oral preparation)

## Oxymetazoline

*Brand Names:* Afrin, Duration, St. Joseph Decongestant for Children

*Description and Uses:* Oxymetazoline is an effective topical nasal decongestant with a somewhat longer duration of action than phenylephrine, ephedrine, and xylometazoline. It has less side effects secondary to stimulation of the nervous system than phenylephrine and ephedrine. There is a significant problem with rebound swelling and inflammation of the nasal passages after withdrawal of the medication. This has led to habituation and prolonged use of the medicine in some individuals. Do *not* use for more than three days in a row.

*Preparations:* Drops: 0.025%, 0.05% concentration. Spray: 0.05% concentration

*Dosage:* INFANTS: See your physician
TODDLERS: 1–2 drops, 0.025% solution in each nostril
SCHOOL AGE: 2–3 drops, 0.025% solution in each nostril
ADOLESCENTS: 2–4 drops, 0.05% solution in each nostril or 2 to 3 squeezes of spray 0.05% concentration in each nostril

*Storage:* Spray and dropper bottle should be discarded after use, for they can become contaminated with bacteria.

*Side Effects:* COMMON: Stinging,* burning,* dryness of the nasal passages,* sneezing*
INFREQUENT: Headache,** sleeplessness,**

dizziness,\*\*\* palpitations (heart skips a beat, or beats fast or irregularly),\*\*\* high blood pressure\*\*\*

*Comments:* To minimize contamination with bacteria, wash the spray tip off with hot water after each usage. Do not share droppers or spray bottles and do not place the dropper directly in the nose.

## Pemoline

*Brand Name:* Cylert

*Description and Uses:* Pemoline is a central nervous system stimulant used as part of the management plan for children with hyperkinetic syndrome. Although pemoline is effective in improving some aspects of this syndrome, long-term effects on learning are inconclusive. In comparison studies with methylphenidate and dextroamphetamine its effects were similar in many respects though not as effective as methylphenidate nor as rapid in onset as either of the two others. Its advantage is that it has no cardiovascular side effects.

*Preparations:* Tablets: 18.75, 37.5, 75 mg. Chewable tablets: 37.5 mg (orange flavor)

*Dosage:* SCHOOL AGE: Initially, one early-morning dose of 37.5 mg increased incrementally until effective. Maximum dose 112.5 mg/daily. May take longer than other drugs to see effects (3 to 4 months)

*Side Effects:* COMMON: Decreased appetite,\*\* insomnia,\*\* weight loss,\*\* growth retardation\*\*
INFREQUENT: Dizziness,\*\*\* headache,\*\*\* skin rash,\*\*\* nausea,\*\*\* depression\*\*\*
RARE: Jaundice\*\*\*

## Penicillin

*Brand Names:* *Penicillin-G*, Falopen, G-Recillin, Hylenta,

Kesso-pen, Novopen-G, P-SO, Penloral, Pentids, Pfizerpen, SK-Penicillin-G, Sugracillin, *Penicillin-V:* Betapen-VK, Compocillin-VK, Ledercillin VK, Nadopen-V, Novopen-V, Penapar VK, PVFK, Repen VK, Robicillin VK, SK-Penicillin VK, Viticillin VK, V-cillin K, VC-K, Veetids

*Description and Uses:* Penicillin is one of the oldest and most dependable antibiotics in medicine. It is used in pediatrics to treat throat infections caused by the streptococcus bacterium (strep throat), skin infections caused by the streptococcus, susceptible urinary tract infections, and in the prevention of the recurrence of rheumatic fever and prevention of heart infections in children with congenital heart disease. Penicillin is available in two forms for oral use, Penicillin-G and Penicillin-V. Penicillin-G is not absorbed as well as Penicillin-V (but is less expensive) in an equal dose, and is reserved for prevention of rheumatic fever and treatment of mild infections. More serious infections and the prevention of heart infection in children with congenital heart disease require the use of Penicillin-V.

*Preparations:* **Penicillin-G:** Suspension, 125 mg (200,000 units), 156 mg, and 250 mg/5 ml. Tablets: 62.5 mg, 125 mg, 156 mg, 250 mg, 3.2 mg, and 500 mg. **Penicillin-V:** Suspension: 125 mg/ml, 125 mg/5 ml, 250 mg/ml, 250 mg/5 ml. Tablets: 125 mg, 250 mg, 500 mg

*Dosage:* *Penicillin-G and Penicillin-V*

    INFANTS: 25–50 mg every 6 hours
    TODDLERS: 100 mg every 6 hours
    SCHOOL AGE: 250 mg every 6 hours
    ADOLESCENTS: 250-500 mg every 6 hours

*Storage:* The oral solutions need to be refrigerated.

*Side Effects:* COMMON: Rash,** diarrhea,** vomiting***
    LESS FREQUENT: Darkening of the tongue (fungal overgrowth)**
    RARE: Blood in urine,*** wheezing,*** itching,*** hives***

*Comments:* Penicillin-G and V need to be taken on an empty stomach. Acidic juices and beverages should not be taken concurrently when taking Penicillin-G.

## Phenobarbital

*Brand Names:* Eskabarb, Luminal

*Description and Uses:* Phenobarbital is a long-acting barbiturate that is one of the most widely used and safest drugs used in the treatment of children's seizures. It is most commonly used as the initial drug in generalized (grand mal) seizures and partial (localized motor or sensory) seizures. Phenobarbital has also been used as a sedative in children; but because of its long action, in addition to the infrequent indications for sedatives at all in children, we do not recommend it for this purpose.

*Preparations:* Drops: 16 mg/ml. Elixir: 20 mg/5 ml. Tablets: 7.5, 15, 30, 60, 90, 100 mg

*Dosage:* INFANTS: 20–30 mg in 1 or 2 divided doses
TODDLERS: 40–60 mg in 1 or 2 divided doses
SCHOOL AGE: 80–120 mg in 1 or 2 divided doses
ADOLESCENTS: 200–300 mg in 1 or 2 divided doses

*Side Effects:* COMMON: Drowsiness,* hyperactivity**
INFREQUENT: Dizziness***
RARE: Fatigue, paleness of skin and lips secondary to anemia***

*Comments:* May be taken with food or mixed with water, milk, or juice.

## Phenylephrine

*Brand Names:* Coricidin, Neo-synephrine, Super Anahist Nasal Spray

*Description and Uses:* Phenylephrine is one of the most widely used topical nasal decongestants. It is an effective short-acting decongestant with less side effects secondary to stimulation of the nervous system than other decongestants such as ephedrine. Like most topical decongestants, prolonged use of phenylephrine can cause rebound swelling and inflammation of the nasal passages after withdrawal of the medication. Do *not* use for more than 3 days in a row.

*Preparations:* Available generically in 0.25% and 1% solutions. Commercially it is available in 0.125%, 0.167%, 0.2%, 0.25%, 0.5% and 1.0% solutions.

*Dosage:* INFANTS: 0.125% solution, 1–2 drops in each nostril
TODDLERS: 0.125% or 0.25% solutions, 1–2 drops in each nostril
SCHOOL AGE: 0.25% solution, 1–2 drops in each nostril
ADOLESCENTS: 0.25% or 0.5% solutions, 1–2 drops in each nostril

*Storage:* Topical nasal decongestant bottles or spray packs should be discarded after use, for the solutions can become quickly contaminated with bacteria.

*Side Effects:* INFREQUENT: Increased activity,* loss of appetite,* sleeplessness,* burning or stinging of the nasal lining,* palpitations (heart skips a beat, beats rapidly or irregularly),*** high blood pressure ***

*Comments:* To minimize the contamination of topical nasal decongestant solutions, rinse the dropper or spray tip in hot water after each use. Do not share droppers or sprayers, and try not to place the dropper in the child's nostril.

### Phenylpropanolamine

*Brand Names:* Available generically; Propadrine

*Description and Uses:* Phenylpropanolamine is one of the most frequently used oral nasal decongestants. It is effective in the treatment of acute rhinitis associated with the common cold, allergic rhinitis, and sinusitis. It has not been documented to be more or less effective than other oral decongestants.

*Preparations:* Capsules: 25 and 50 mg. Elixir: 20 mg/15 ml. Phenylpropanolamine is also a part of numerous cold medicines in amounts ranging from 15 mg to 100 mg for tablets and from 5 mg to 20 mg for liquids.

*Dosage:*  INFANTS: 2.5–5 mg 3–4 times a day
TODDLERS: 5–10 mg 3–4 times per day
SCHOOL AGE: 10–15 mg 3–4 times per day
ADOLESCENTS: 15–25 mg 4–6 times per day

*Storage:*  May be stored without refrigeration

*Side Effects:*  COMMON: Hyperactivity,* nervousness,* sleeplessness,* loss of appetite*
INFREQUENT: Dizziness,*** palpitations (heart skips a beat),*** nausea and vomiting,*** high blood pressure***

*Comments:* Phenylpropanolamine is also prescribed as a diet suppressant in adults. In this form, it has been abused as an "upper." The last daily dose should be taken several hours before bedtime to avoid trouble sleeping.


## Phenytoin

*Brand Name:* Dilantin

*Description and Uses:* Phenytoin is a commonly used anticonvulsant in children for the treatment of generalized seizures, and focal motor seizures (seizures confined to a particular part of the brain). Although phenytoin is an effective anticonvulsant it is rarely the initial drug used in children because of a significant incidence of side effects. Phenytoin has also been used to treat migraine headaches in older children. Its efficacy for this condition is unproved.

*Preparations:*   Suspension: 30 mg/5 ml, 125 mg/5 ml. Tablets: 30, 50 mg. Capsules: 30 mg, 100 mg (extended)

*Dosage:*   INFANTS: 12.5–15 mg twice a day
TODDLERS: 25–35 mg twice a day
SCHOOL AGE: 50–75 mg twice a day. May be given as one daily dose in extended capsule form.
ADOLESCENTS: 75–150 mg twice a day. May be given as one daily dose in extended capsule form.

*Side Effects:*   COMMON: Overgrowth of the gums,* overgrowth of hair,* ataxia***
INFREQUENT: Skin rash,*** double vision***
RARE: Swollen lymph gland,** fatigue and yellow jaundice secondary to hepatitis,*** severe blistering skin rash,*** decreased production of blood,*** pallor and fatigue secondary to anemia,*** darkening of urine***

*Comments:*   The oral suspension needs to be well shaken to avoid overdosage with a concentration of suspension at the bottom of the bottle. The overgrowth of the gums can be avoided to some extent by oral hygiene (thoroughly brushing and flossing of teeth). Generic preparations are not equivalent to Dilantin and should *not* be used interchangably. Only capsules labelled "extended" can be used for once daily dosing. May be given with meals to decrease stomach upset.

## Prednisone

*Brand Names:*   Deltasone, Meticorten, Orasone

*Description and Uses:*   Prednisone is a member of a class of drugs known as steroids. Steroids in the body are manufactured by the adrenal gland. When synthetic steroids, such as prednisone, are administered for therapeutic reasons, it is possible to suppress the normal functioning of the adrenal gland. Generally this occurs after several weeks. In therapeutic dosages prednisone is effective in treating a number of conditions. It also creates numerous other predictable problems, which are not true side effects but which are expected because of this drug's biochemical and physiologic properties. Though prednisone is highly effective, it must always be carefully weighed because of its numerous side effects.

In this book, prednisone has been discussed principally in the treatment of severe asthma. Parents may also on occasion be given a one-week prescription for prednisone or other closely related steroid to treat severe contact dermatitis (poison oak or ivy) or a severe allergic reaction or insect bite, or to control a particularly severe bout of allergic rhinitis.

For children receiving chronic prednisone, administration on an every-other-day regimen results in less pituitary and adrenal gland suppression. This in turn minimizes growth suppression and obesity.

*Preparations:*   Tablets: 1, 2.5, 5, 10, 20, 50 mg

*Dosage:*   Individually determined according to type of illness.

*Side Effects:*   The frequency of these pharmacologic effects depends on dosage and frequency of administration as well as on the individual patient. At a high enough dosage, all are common: gastric irritation and bleeding,** growth suppression,** weight gain,** headache,** dizziness,** increased infections,** personality changes,** fluid retention**

*Comments:*   Prednisone can reactivate tuberculosis. Always have your child tuberculin tested before beginning prednisone. During severe stresses children may require additional steroids, for their adrenal glands may be suppressed and unable to respond normally. May take with food to decrease stomach upset. Do *not* stop using this medicine without first checking with your doctor. Your doctor may want to gradually reduce the amount you are using in order to avoid serious side effects.

## Prochlorperazine

*Brand Name:* Compazine

*Description and Uses:* Prochlorperazine is a member of a class of drugs known as phenothiazines. It is effective in treating the nausea and vomiting that accompany radiation or chemotherapy, toxins, and postoperative states. It is not recommended for use when vomiting accompanies gastroenteritis.

*Preparations:* Solution: 10 mg/ml. Syrup: 5 mg/teaspoon. Suppositories: 2.5, 5, 25 mg. Capsules: 10, 15, 30, 75 mg. Tablets: 5, 10 mg

*Dosage:* INFANTS AND TODDLERS: Not recommended
SCHOOL AGE: 2.5 mg suppository 3 or 4 times daily
ADOLESCENTS: 5 mg suppository 3 or 4 times daily

*Side Effects:* INFREQUENT: Drowsiness,* dry mouth,* dizziness,** restlessness,** constipation,** gait disturbances,*** slurred speech,*** blurred vision,*** skin rash,*** menstrual periods stop***
RARE: Weakness upon standing,*** gall bladder obstruction,*** gastroenteritis,*** movement disorders***

*Comments:* The side effects seen with the use of prochlorperazine may resemble symptoms seen with serious central nervous system diseases. Prochlorperazine should be used cautiously and only if the origin of the vomiting is known and other measures (dietary) have failed.

## Promethazine

*Brand Names:* Phenergan, Remsed

*Description and Uses:* Promethazine has been used in children to treat nausea and vomiting (motion sickness), as an antihistamine for allergies and colds (it is frequently combined with codeine to treat the cough of a cold), and as a sedative. It is effective in the treatment of motion sickness, but less effective in the treatment of nausea and vomiting caused by an illness or drugs. It is an effective antihistamine in allergy, and questionably effective in the treatment of the runny nose of a cold. Because of its marked sedative effect, its use is usually limited to before bedtime.

*Preparations:*  Syrup: 6.25 mg and 25 mg/5 ml. Tablets: 12.5 mg, 25 mg, 50 mg

*Dosage:*  *For nausea and vomiting:*     *For sedative:*

| | |
|---|---|
| INFANTS: 1.25–2.5 mg every 4–6 hours | INFANTS: 2.5–5.0 mg as needed |
| TODDLERS: 2.5 mg every 4–6 hours | TODDLERS: 5.0–10 mg as needed |
| SCHOOL AGE: 10 mg every 4–6 hours | SCHOOL AGE: 10–20 mg as needed |
| ADOLESCENTS: 12.5–25 mg every 4–6 hours | ADOLESCENTS: 20–40 mg as needed |

*For cold or allergy:*

INFANTS: Not indicated
TODDLERS: 2.5 mg every 4–6 hours
SCHOOL AGE: 5 mg every 4–6 hours
ADOLESCENTS: 6.25–12.5 mg every 4–6 hours

*Storage:*  Promethazine syrup and tablets should be kept out of the light and extreme heat and cold. The syrup does not need to be refrigerated.

*Side Effects:*  COMMON: Drowsiness,* dryness of mouth, nose, and throat*
LESS FREQUENT: Nervousness,** insomnia,** dizziness,** skin rash***
RARE: Frequent and/or serious infection (decreased production of white blood cells)***

*Comments:*  To prevent motion sickness, promethazine should be taken twice a day.

## Pseudoephedrine

*Brand Names:*   Afrinol-Symptom 2, Novafed, Sudafed

*Description and Uses:*   Pseudoephedrine is an effective oral and nasal decongestant that is a common ingredient in many cold remedies. It is similar to ephedrine in effectiveness, but is thought to possibly have less nervous-system side effects.

*Preparations:*   Tablets: 30, 60 mg. Capsules: time released, 120 mg. Syrup: 30 mg/5 ml

*Dosage:*   INFANTS: 6–10 mg every 6 hours
TODDLERS: 10–15 mg every 6 hours
SCHOOL AGE: 15–40 mg every 6 hours
ADOLESCENTS: 40–60 mg every 6 hours

*Storage:*   May be stored without refrigeration

*Side Effects:*   COMMON: Increased activity,* sleeplessness,* decreased appetite*
INFREQUENT: Dizziness,*** palpitations (heart skips a beat or beats rapidly),*** high blood pressure***

*Comments:*   To prevent sleeplessness take last daily dose several hours before bedtime. May take with food.

## Pyrantel Pamoate

*Brand Name:*   Antiminth

*Description and Uses:*   Pyrantel pamoate is an effective antibiotic for the treatment of roundworm and pinworm. It is almost 100% effective with just one dose in the treatment of roundworm (it is the drug of choice for this condition) and 90–100% effective with one dose in the treatment of pinworm (it is, along with mebendazole, the drug of choice for this condition). It is also 90% effective in the treatment of most cases of hookworm.

*Preparation:*   Suspension: 250 mg/5 ml (caramel flavor)

*Dosage:*   *Pinworm and roundworm:*
INFANTS: 65–100 mg in 1 dose
TODDLERS: 100–150 mg in 1 dose
SCHOOL AGE: 150–500 mg in 1 dose
ADOLESCENTS: 500–1000 mg in 1 dose

*Hookworm:*
INFANTS: 65–100 mg every day for 3 days
TODDLERS: 100–150 mg every day for 3 days
SCHOOL AGE: 150–500 mg every day for 3 days
ADOLESCENTS: 500–1000 mg every day for 3 days

*Storage:*   Pyrantel pamoate may be stored without refrigeration.

*Side Effects:*   INFREQUENT: Diarrhea,** vomiting,** abdominal pain**
RARE: Drowsiness,** headache,*** dizziness,*** rash,*** inflammation of the liver (look for fatigue, yellowing of the skin, loss of appetite)***

*Comments:*   Pyrantel pamoate may be taken before, with, or after meals.


## Pyrethins

*Brand Names:*   A-200 Pyrinate, RID, TISIT, TISIT Blue, Triple X

*Description and Uses:*   These substances, derived from the chrysanthemum plant, appear to be effective in the treatment of head, body, and pubic lice. The medications are available without a prescription. Their effectiveness with respect to other antilice medicines has not been evaluated.

*Preparations:*   Pyrethins are available in a lotion shampoo or a gel (the gel is used for head and pubic hair regions).

*Dosage:*   The pyrethin preparation should be applied over the affected region, and rinsed off after 10 minutes. Application may need to be repeated again, but should not be repeated within a 24-hour period.

*Storage:*  Pyrethin preparations may be stored without refrigeration.

*Comments:*  Extreme care should be taken to keep pyrethin preparations out of the eyes, for they may cause extreme irritation and ulceration of the cornea.

## Quinacrine

*Brand Name:*  Atabrine

*Description and Uses:*  Quinacrine is an effective antibiotic against the protozoa *Giardia* and has been one of the drugs of choice (along with metronidazole) in the treatment of giardiasis. Frequent side effects (see below) and decreasing concern over the cancer-causing potential of metronidazole have caused many physicians to choose metronidazole over quinacrine as the drug of choice for giardiasis.

*Preparation:*  Tablets: 100 mg

*Dosage:*  INFANTS: 15 mg 3 times a day
TODDLERS: 25 mg 3 times a day
SCHOOL AGE: 50 mg 3 times a day
ADOLESCENTS: 100 mg 3 times a day

*Storage:*  May be stored without refrigeration

*Side Effects:*  COMMON: Nausea,** vomiting,** temporary yellowish discoloration of the skin**
INFREQUENT: Dizziness,*** marked changes in behavior***
RARE: Decreased production of elements of the blood (look for easy bruising, frequent or serious infections, or pallor),*** destruction of the liver (look for fatigue, yellow jaundice, vomiting, loss of appetite)***

*Comments:*  Quinacrine has a very bitter taste. Tablets may be crushed and mixed with jam or honey. It is best taken after meals followed by a full glass of water, tea, or fruit juice.

## Salicylic Acid/Lactic Acid Mixture

*Brand Name:* Duofilm, Salactic Film

*Description and Uses:* This combination of acids is an effective way of treating warts at home. It works by softening the surface of the skin where the virus that causes the wart resides. The skin can then be separated away. This combination is effective 60–80% of the time with most common warts within a 12-week period. Treatment of plantar warts (warts on the bottom of the foot) may require a longer period of time.

*Preparation:* 16.7% salicylic acid and 16.7% lactic acid in flexible collodion

*Dosage:* This preparation should be applied to the wart nightly. The wart should be rubbed or scraped gently with a pumice stone or emory board prior to application.

*Storage:* May be stored without refrigeration

*Side Effects:* INFREQUENT: Acute ulceration and inflammation can occur with prolonged use***

## Selenium Sulfide

*Brand Names:* Exsel, Iosel 250, Selsun, Selsun Blue

*Description and Uses:* Selenium sulfide is one of the most effective medicated shampoos in the treatment of dandruff and seborrhea of the scalp.

*Preparations:* Shampoo, lotion: 1% (nonprescription), 2.5% (prescription). Cream: 1% (nonprescription)

*Dosage:* One or two teaspoons are applied to the wet scalp

(and worked into a lather if it is a shampoo), left on the scalp for 3–5 minutes, and then rinsed off. For extensive cases the treatment can be repeated. This treatment should be used 1–3 times per week.

*Storage:* May be stored without refrigeration

*Side Effects:* It may increase normal hair loss.** When applied to normal skin, selenium sulfide has almost no side effects. If the skin is red, raw, or irritated, selenium sulfide may increase the irritation and should not be used.***

*Comments:* Care should be taken to avoid contact with eyes during application. Do not take internally. Shake well before use and wash hands after use.


### Steroids (Topical)

*Brand Names:* Available generically; *dexamethosone sodium phosphate:* Decadron; *methylprednisolone:* Medrol; *flumethasone pivalate:* Locorten; *desonide:* Tridesilon; *triamcinolone:* Aristocort, Kenalog; *flurandrenolide:* Cordran; *betamethasone valerate:* Valisone; *halcinonide:* Halog; *fluocinonide:* Lidex, Topsyn; *desoximetasone:* Topicort

*Description and Uses:* About one-half of all drugs prescribed for use on the skin are steroids. Steroids are effective agents in combating inflammation and therefore they are useful against a number of both chronic and acute skin conditions. They are commonly used against atopic dermatitis (eczema), seborrhea dermatitis, and allergic contact dermatitis. They may also be recommended for small patches of poison ivy or oak, although this use remains controversial. Steroids are not useful for skin problems such as acne, or rashes secondary to infection such as impetigo. They may occasionally be used to hasten healing in a particularly severe or recalcitrant form of diaper rash.

*Preparations:* A variety of steroids are available that vary considerably in potency. In addition, preparations are available as creams, ointments, and lotions. In general, for a given preparation, gels are the strongest, followed by ointments, creams, and lotions. The following is a sampling of topical steroids ranked according to equivalent classes of potency, the strongest being listed first. Class I: Halog cream 0.1%, Lidex cream and ointment 0.05%; class II: Valisone ointment and lotion 0.1%; class III: Synalar ointment 0.025%, Cordran ointment 0.05%, Kenalog ointment 0.1%, Aristocort ointment 0.01%; class IV: Kenalog creme 0.1%, Synalar creme 0.025%, Kenalog lotion 0.025%; class V: Locorten creme 0.03%, Desonide creme 0.05%; class VI: 1% hydrocortisone cream

*Dosage:* Will vary according to condition being treated as well as area of body. In general, lower dosage preparations are used for the face, skin folds, and sensitive areas around the groin; more potent steroids and preparations are used on the palms and soles.

*Side Effects:* Depend on potency of preparation as well as length of usage. Suppression of the adrenal gland is seldom seen if usage is less than one month.
    INFREQUENT: Skin thinning, acne
    RARE: Skin color changes, adrenal suppression (obesity, acne, increased blood pressure)

*Comments:* All preparations should be kept away from the eyes—glaucoma may result.

## Sulfacetamide Eye Drops

*Brand Names:* Bleph-10, -30, Cetamide, Sodium Sulamyd, Sulfacel-15, Vasosulf

*Description and Uses:* Sulfacetamide is an antibiotic that can shorten the course of conjunctivitis caused by bacterial or chlamydial infections. It is the first-line drug for topical treatment of conjunctivitis in infants and children when non-viral causes are suspected.

*Preparations:* Solution or suspension: 100–300 mg/ml. Ointment: 100–300 mg/gm

*Dosage:* Drops may be administered every 2 hours. Ointment is effective for a longer period of time but obscures vision. It should be administered only at night.

*Side Effects:* INFREQUENT: Transient burning or stinging*
RARE: Severe skin reaction***

Should not be used if child has known sensitivity to sulfa drugs.

*Comments:* After application of the ointment your vision may be blurred for a few minutes.


### Sulfisoxazole

*Brand Names:* Gantrisin, J-Sol, Lipo-gantrisin, Rosoxol, SK-Soxazole, Sulfalar

*Description and Uses:* Sulfisoxazole is an antibiotic that is one member of a group of drugs called sulfa drugs. It is the most commonly prescribed sulfa drug in children, and is used primarily for treatment of urinary tract infections, and in combination with erythromycin (see Pediazole) for treatment of middle-ear infections. Sulfisoxazole is an effective first-line drug for treatment of urinary tract infection in children. It is used as a second-line drug in the treatment of otitis media, for children who are allergic to ampicillin (amoxicillin) or when the offending bacteria may be resistant to ampicillin (this happens 2–3% of the time). If it is used to treat middle-ear infections, it should be used in combination with penicillin or erythromycin.

*Preparations:* Tablet: 450, 500 mg. Suspension: 500 mg/5 ml

*Dosage:* INFANTS: 1.0 g in 4 divided doses
TODDLERS: 2.25 g in 4 divided doses
PRE-SCHOOL AGE: 3.0 g in 4 divided doses
ADOLESCENTS: 4.0 g in 4 divided doses

*Storage:* Suspension should be refrigerated—shake well before using

*Side Effects:* Common: Stomach upset (nausea and vomiting),** diarrhea**

INFREQUENT: Rash,*** headaches,*** lethargy***

RARE: Inflammation of nerves (pain in limbs or other body parts),*** psychotic behavior,*** decreased production of blood products (evident as unusual bruising, serious infections, or easy fatigue),*** inflammation of the liver (evident as listlessness or yellow jaundice)***

*Comments:* Should not be taken by nursing mothers of small infants, or by children with a known allergy to any sulfa drug. Best if taken on an empty stomach.

### Terbutaline Sulfate

*Brand Names:* Brethine, Bricanyl

*Description and Uses:* A newer bronchodilator from the adrenergic class that is very selective in causing bronchodilation. Terbutaline sulfate has very few cardiac side effects and is being used widely as an alternative to epinephrine injections. It is also available in an oral form. Although there are no inhalers, it can be administered by a nebulizer.

*Preparations:* Tablets: 2.5, 5 mg

*Dosage:* SCHOOL AGE: 1.25 mg 3 times a day

ADOLESCENTS: 2.5 mg 3 times a day; may be gradually increased to 5 mg 3 times a day

*Side Effects:* COMMON: Muscle tremor**

INFREQUENT: Dizziness,*** nervousness,*** palpitations,*** fatigue,*** ringing in ears,*** nausea and vomiting***

*Comments:* Because of limited experience with children, terbutaline sulfate is currently not widely used for children under 12. Its relative safety makes us believe that its use will increase in coming years. May take with meals.


## Tetracycline

*Brand Names:* Achromycin, Achromycin V, Bristacycline, Centent, Cyclopar, Fed-mycin, G-mycim, Maytrey, Paltet, Panmycin, Retot, Robitet, Roy-cycline, SK-tetracycline, Sumycin, T-250, Tetrachel, Tetracycn, Tetrey

*Description and Uses:* Because tetracycline is incorporated into the bones and teeth of rapidly growing children and may affect bone and teeth development, causing discoloration of teeth, there is almost no reason to use tetracycline in children under the age of eight years. The most common uses are the treatment of acne in adolescents, in which it is an effective adjunct to topical antiacne therapy. It is also used in the treatment of venereal disease in adolescents. Tetracycline is a frequently prescribed antibiotic for treatment of respiratory and urinary tract infections in adults, but it is rarely the drug of choice in older children and adolescents.

*Preparations:* Capsules: 250, 500 mg. Syrup: 125 mg/15 ml

*Dosage:* OLDER CHILDREN: 250 mg every 6 hours
ADOLESCENTS: 250–500 mg every 6 hours (venereal disease and acne have specific treatment regimens; see Chapter 26, Acne, and consult your physician)

*Storage:* May be stored at room temperature

*Side Effects:* COMMON: Tetracycline should not be prescribed in children under the age of 8, as it may cause disturbances in the growth of bones and teeth, and discoloration of the teeth. Other common side effects include upset stomach (nausea, vomiting, heart burn),** diarrhea,** photosensitivity—redness of skin exposed to sun***

INFREQUENT: Sores on mouth or tongue,** inflammation of the gut (evident as cramps, diarrhea, or blood in the toilet bowl)***

RARE: Serious allergic reactions (low blood pressure or shock and wheezing),*** hives,*** decreased production of clotting substances in the blood platelets (evident as easy bruising)***

*Comments:* If possible, tetracycline should be taken one hour before, or two hours after a meal for maximum effectiveness. Avoid the use of milk, antacids, and iron preparations when taking tetracycline.

## Tetracycline—Topical

*Brand Name:* Topicycline

*Description and Uses:* This preparation is a topical antibiotic used for treatment of acne, generally only after other topical methods have failed. It is not quite as effective as oral tetracycline, but not all patients can tolerate or are willing to take daily oral medicine.

*Preparation:* Powder and diluent reconstitutes to 2.2 mg/ml

*Dosage:* 0.5–1 ml of prepared solution 2 times a day

*Side Effects:* COMMON: Stinging sensation when applying*

*Comments:* Topical tetracycline often stains the skin yellow and fluoresces under black lights. These properties make it less desirable than other topical antibiotics.

## Theophylline and Aminophylline

*Brand Names:* *Theophylline, tablets and capsules:* Bronkodyl 100, 200 mg; Elixophyllin 100, 200 mg; Slo-Phyllin 100,

200 mg; Somophyllin–T 100, 200, 250 mg; Theolair 125, 250 mg; Theophyl–225, 225 mg; Theophyl-chewable 100 mg. *Oral solutions:* Bronkodyl; Elixicon (nonalcoholic) 100 mg/5 ml; Elixophyllin (alcoholic) 27 mg/5 ml; Slo-Phyllin 80, 27 mg/5 ml; Somophyllin Theolair 27 mg/5 ml; Theophyl 37.5 mg/5 ml; Theoclear 80, 27 mg/5 ml; Theospan 27 mg/5 ml. *Timed release tablets or capsules:* Elixophyllin–SR 125, 250 mg; Slo-Phyllin Gyrocaps 60, 125, 250 mg; Sustaire 100, 300 mg; TheoDur 100, 200, 300 mg; Theolair SR 250, 500 mg; Theophyl–SR, 125, 250 mg

*Aminophylline* consists of 85% theophylline and 15% ethylenediamine. It is available generically or as Somophyllin.

*Description and Uses:* Theophylline is a drug of the xanthine class that effectively opens the bronchial passages. It is the most commonly used drug for treating asthma. It has several other properties that make it effective in treating breathing problems in newborns caused by immature nervous systems.

*Preparations:* See Brand Names.

*Dosage:* There is considerable individual variation in the dosage of theophylline necessary to give a safe blood level that effectively opens the air passages. Younger children often require higher dosages per pound of body weight than do adults. Your physician will probably take blood level tests to help individualize dosing.

| *Every 6 hours* | *Every 8–12 hours, timed-release preparations* |
| --- | --- |
| INFANTS: 25 mg | INFANTS: 30 mg every 8 hrs |
| TODDLERS: 50 mg | TODDLERS: 60 mg every 8 hrs |
| SCHOOL AGE: 100 mg | SCHOOL AGE: 200 mg every 12 hours |
| ADOLESCENTS: 150 mg | ADOLESCENTS: 300 mg every 12 hours |

*Side Effects:* COMMON: Stomach aches,** headache,** dizziness,** irritability,** nausea,** vomiting**

LESS FREQUENT: Insomnia,*** persistent vomiting,*** agitation***

RARE: Vomiting blood,*** fever,*** convulsions,*** heart irregularities***

*Comments:* The number of theophylline preparations is increasing each year. Not all the preparations are equally effective. Therefore exercise caution if your physician changes preparations.

Many preparations are available as both timed-release and standard preparations. Make sure that you are giving the appropriate medicine. Timed-release preparations are usually used when children take theophylline as a daily medicine. If your child is instructed to take theophylline only when an asthma attack begins, a standard preparation will achieve therapeutic levels more rapidly than will timed-release preparations. Aminophylline preparations offer no advantage over theophylline; 15% more aminophylline (for equivalent effect) must be given as it consists of 85% theophylline. May be taken with meals to minimize upset stomach.

**Tolnaftate**

*Brand Names:* Aftate, Tinactin

*Description and Uses:* Tolnaftate is an antifungal drug that is effective against most fungus infections of the skin. Unlike many of the other topical antifungals, tolnaftate has no activity against *Candida* or yeast infections, and is not useful in diaper rashes and vaginitis.

*Preparations:* Gel: 1%. Powder: 1% (aerosol). Liquid (aerosol): 1%. Solution: 1%. Cream: 1% concentration. Powder: 1%

*Dosage:* One or two drops of solution, or a thin layer of cream, are applied two or three times a week. Resolution of the infection usually takes place in 2–3 weeks, but may take up to 4–6 weeks.

*Storage:* May be stored without refrigeration

*Side Effects:* No documented side effects have been reported

*Comments:* Tolnaftate is not effective against fungus infections of the hair, nails, palms, or soles.

## Tretinoin

*Brand Name:* Retin–A

*Description and Uses:* An effective agent in controlling acne. It acts by increasing skin peeling, which prevents blocking of sebaceous glands.

*Preparations:* Cream: 0.05, 0.1%. Gel: 0.01, 0.025%. Liquid swabs: 0.5% concentration.

*Dosage:* Nightly application to involved area. Start with lowest concentration. Avoid make-up, coarse soaps, excess sun. If redness or peeling of skin are noticed, apply less frequently. Should not be used in patients with eczema. Avoid contact with eyes, mouth, and nose. Do not use immediately after shower.

*Side Effects:* COMMON: Peeling, redness, and stinging commonly occur*
LESS FREQUENT: Peeling and redness longer than 3 weeks**

*Comments:* Good results are often not noted for three months. Because of its irritating quality, some skin may look worse for several weeks. Proper usage results in only minimal peeling. Effectiveness can be judged after 4 months of regular usage. May be used in combination with benzoyl peroxide. Avoid using tretinoin with abrasive soaps as this may lead to excessive redness. Thoroughly dry the skin prior to applying.

## Triaminic

*Combination Drug:* Pheniramine, phenylpropanolamine, pyrilamine

*Description and Uses:* Antihistamines (pheniramine and pyrilamine) as well as an adrenergic sympathomimetic (phenylpropanolamine) have a drying effect on the membranes of the nose. Although they may be used together for the relief of this symptom during a cold, there is no evidence that they are effective in preventing or treating ear infections. We do not advise this type of combination drug as a means of counteracting the side effects of the individual components (nervousness and insomnia for phenylpropanolamine, and drowsiness for the antihistamines).

*Preparations:* Syrup: Phenylpropanolamine 12.5 mg, pheniramine 6.25 mg, pyrilamine 6.25 mg/5 ml. Oral infant drops: Phenylpropanolamine 20 mg, pheniramine 10 mg, pyrilamine 10 mg/1 ml. Tablets: Phenylpropanolamine 50 mg, pheniramine 25 mg, pyrilamine 25 mg timed-release tablets

*Dosage:*   INFANTS: Consult physician for individual dosage
TODDLERS: 1 teaspoonful 3 times daily
SCHOOL AGE: 1–2 teaspoons syrup 3 to 4 times daily
ADOLESCENTS: 2–3 teaspoons 3 to 4 times daily/2 tablets twice daily

*Side Effects:* *See* phenylpropanolamine; pyrilamine: same as other antihistamines, but drowsiness occurs less frequently


### Trimethobenzamide

*Brand Name:* Tigan

*Description and Uses:* This drug is used to reduce frequent vomiting. It is also effective in relieving nausea, but it has little or no effect in reducing dizziness or treating motion sickness. It acts by inhibiting the vomiting center in the brain.

*Preparations:* Capsules: 100, 250 mg. Suppositories: 100 (pediatric), 200 mg

*Dosage:* INFANTS: Not for newborns; ¼ pediatric suppository 3 to 4 times daily
TODDLERS: ½ pediatric suppository 3 to 4 times
daily
SCHOOL AGE: 1 pediatric suppository 3 to 4 times
daily
ADOLESCENTS: 200 mg suppository 3 to 4 times
daily

*Side Effects:* INFREQUENT: Dry mouth,* headache,**
drowsiness,*** blurred vision,*** dizziness,*** skin rash,*** diarrhea***
RARE: Convulsions,*** gait disturbance,*** liver problems***

*Comments:* Trimethobenzamide suppositories are used frequently in children receiving radiation therapy. Although
they are effective in gastroenteritis, they have numerous side
effects and should be used only when other dietary strategies
have failed.

## Trimethoprim Sulfamethoxazole

*Brand Names:* Bactrim, Septra

*Description and Uses:* Trimethoprim sulfamethoxazole is an
effective combination of two antiobiotics that attack bacteria
in two different ways. It is effective in the treatment of urinary tract infections, prevention of urinary tract infections
(prophylaxis), otitis media, and respiratory infections caused
by bacteria. It is the first-line drug for prevention of urinary
tract infections. Physicians are increasingly using this drug as
the first-line drug for otitis media. It is as effective as ampicillin (and in some cases effective against bacteria resistant to
ampicillin), but it may have a higher rate of side effects. It
has the additional advantages of a twice-a-day dosage, and
storage without refrigeration.

*Preparations:* Suspension: 40 mg trimethoprim/200 mg sulfamethoxazole per 5 ml. Tablets: 80 mg trimethoprim/400 mg

sulfamethoxazole, and 160 mg trimethoprim/800 mg sulfamethoxazole (double-strength—DS)

*Dosage:*    INFANTS: ½–1 tsp
                TODDLERS: 1–2 tsp
                SCHOOL AGE: 2–3 tsp; 1–1½ tablets
                ADOLESCENTS: 4 tsp; 2 tablets (1 DS tablet)

*Storage:*    Suspension may be stored without refrigeration.

*Side Effects:*    COMMON: Stomach upset,** vomiting,** diarrhea**
                INFREQUENT: Skin rash,*** headache,*** lethargy***
                RARE: Inflammation of kidney,*** psychotic behavior,*** decreased production of blood products,*** inflammation of the liver (evident as listlessness, yellow jaundice)***

*Comments:*    This drug combination should not be taken by nursing mothers of newborn infants. Do not give this medicine if your child is allergic to any sulfa medicine. Take on an empty stomach. It has a bitter after taste.

## Tripelennamine

*Brand Names:*    PBZ citrate, PBZ–SR, Pyribenzamine HC1

*Description and Uses:*    Tripelennamine is an antihistamine that is effective in the treatment of hay fever (seasonal allergic rhinitis). Of children with this condition, 75–90% will receive some symptomatic relief with this antihistamine. It is also effective in the treatment of an allergic "stuffy nose" (non-seasonal allergic rhinitis), but has not been proved effective in the treatment of the common cold. It is a member of a class of antihistamines called ethylenediamines, whose major side effects are dizziness and sedation. It is midway between diphenhydramine (Benadryl) and chlorpheniramine in the incidence of drowsiness. It has not been shown to be more or less effective than other antihistamines in the treatment of the above mentioned conditions. Some physicians feel that it is not as effective as other types of antihistamines in the treatment of hives; however, it can be effective in the treatment of other itchy skin disorders.

*Preparations:*  Tablets: 25, 50 mg; timed-release, 50, 100 mg. Elixir: 375 mg/15ml

*Dosage:*  Regular Form:
 INFANTS: 7.5–10 mg every 6 hours
 TODDLERS: 10–15 mg every 6 hours
 SCHOOL AGE: 15–25 mg every 6 hours
 ADOLESCENTS: 25–50 mg every 6 hours

 Timed-release form:
 SCHOOL AGE: 50 mg every 8–12 hours
 ADOLESCENTS: 100 mg every 8–12 hours

*Storage:*  May be stored without refrigeration

*Side Effects:*  COMMON: Drowsiness,* difficulty concentrating,* nausea and vomiting***
 INFREQUENT: Increased activity,* insomnia,* dizziness,** tremors,** palpitations (heart skipping a beat, or beating fast or irregularly)**
 RARE: Frequent urination,** decreased production of blood products (look for easy bruising, or frequent or serious infections),*** confusion,*** headaches,*** chills***

*Comments:*  Because of the frequent behavioral disturbances associated with the administration of antihistamines, care should be taken in giving this medicine to children before school, skateboard riding, roller skating, bicycle riding, or operation of a potentially dangerous tool or toy. May be taken with meals to decrease stomach upset. Do not break, crush, or chew the time-release forms.

## Tripolidine

*Brand Name:* Actidil

*Description and Uses:* Tripolidine is an antihistamine effective in the treatment of hay fever. Of children with this condition, 75–90% will receive some symptomatic relief from this medication. Tripolidine is also effective in the treatment of allergic "stuffy nose" (nonseasonal allergic rhinitis), but it has not been proved effective in the treatment of the common cold. It has not been shown more or less effective than other antihistamines in the treatment of these conditions. It may be less effective than other types of antihistamines in the treatment of hives, but it has been used for other itchy skin conditions. Tripolidine is a member of a class of antihistamines (alkylamines) that has the lowest incidence of associated drowsiness. This makes it a useful antihistamine for daytime use.

*Preparations:* Tablets: 2.5 mg. Syrup: 1.25 mg/5ml

*Dosage:* INFANTS: 0.3–0.6 mg every 6 hours
TODDLERS: 0.6–1.25 mg every 6 hours
SCHOOL AGE: 1.25–2.5 mg every 6 hours
ADOLESCENTS: 2.5 mg every 6 hours

*Storage:* May be stored without refrigeration

*Side Effects:* COMMON: Drowsiness,* inability to concentrate*
INFREQUENT: Increased activity,* insomnia,* dizziness,*** nausea and vomiting,*** palpitations (heart skips a beat, beats fast or irregularly)***
RARE: Frequent urination,** decreased production of blood products*** (look for easy bruising, frequent or serious infections), headaches,*** confusion,*** chills***

*Comments:* Because of the frequent behavioral disturbances associated with the administration of antihistamines, care should be taken in giving this medication to your child before school, skateboarding, rollerskating, bicycle riding, or operation of a potentially dangerous tool or toy. May take with food to decrease stomach upset.

## Vitamin A, C, D Supplement

*Brand Name:*  Tri-Vi-Sol; Tri-Vi-Flor is Tri-Vi-Sol with fluoride

*Description and Uses:*  The only routine indication for vitamin supplementation in children is for infants being exclusively breast fed. Children may experience isolated deficiencies that should be treated with a therapeutic amount of the particular deficient vitamin. In areas where water supplies are not naturally or chemically fluoridated to give 0.3 ppm fluoride concentration, infants (birth to 2 years) should receive 0.25 mg of fluoride, toddlers (2–3 years) should receive 0.5 mg, and children over 3 years, 1.0 mg. Tri-Vi-Flor contains 0.5 mg fluoride and should not be used in infants less than six months. Tri-Vi-Sol is also available with iron.

*Preparation:*  Tri-Vi-Sol drops: each ml contains 1500 units vitamin A, 400 units vitamin D, and 35 mg ascorbic acid (vitamin C)

*Dosage:*  One dropperful (0.6 ml) daily for breast-fed infants

*Side Effects:*  None in proper dosage

*Comments:*  Be sure to read Chapter 11, Infant Formulas, and Chapter 12 on vitamins and minerals.

## Xylometazoline

*Brand Names:*  Dristan Long Lasting, 4-Way Long Acting, Neo-synephrine II, Once-A-Day, Otrivin Hydrochloride, Sine-off, Sinex Long Acting, Sinutab Long Lasting Sinus Spray

*Description and Uses:* Xylometazoline is a topical nasal decongestant effective for temporary relief of nasal congestion. It is similar to oxymetazoline, but has a shorter duration of action. Compared to other antihistamines, it has less side effects secondary to stimulation of the nervous system, but it does have a significant problem with rebound swelling and inflammation of the nasal passages after withdrawal of the medicine.

*Preparations:* Drops: 0.05, 0.1% concentration. Spray: 0.1% concentration.

*Dosage:*  INFANTS: See your physician
TODDLERS: 1–2 drops, 0.05% solution each nostril every 8–10 hours
SCHOOL AGE: 2–3 drops in each nostril every 8–10 hours
ADOLESCENTS: 2–3 drops, 0.1% solution in each nostril, or 1–2 inhalations of nasal spray in each nostril every 8–10 hours

*Storage:* Spray containers and dropper bottles should be discarded after use, for they can become contaminated with bacteria over time.

*Side Effects:*  COMMON: Local stinging,* burning,* sneezing,* and dryness of the nose*
INFREQUENT: Headache,*** insomnia,*** palpitations (heart skips a beat or beats rapidly or irregularly),*** dizziness***

*Comments:* To minimize bacterial contamination, wash the spray tip with hot water after each use. Do not share droppers or spray bottles, and do not place the dropper directly in the nose.


## Zinc Pyrithione

*Brand Names:* Breck One Shampoo, Danex Shampoo, Head and Shoulders Shampoo, Zincon Shampoo

*Description and Uses:* Zinc pyrithione is an effective medicated shampoo for the treatment of dandruff and seborrhea of the scalp.

*Preparations:* Shampoo: 1%, 2% concentration

*Dosage:* One or two teaspoons of shampoo are worked into the wet scalp and left for up to 5 minutes before thoroughly rinsing off. The application is then repeated. The treatment should be done once or twice weekly.

*Side Effects:* There are no known side effects when applied as directed to normal skin and hair

*Comments:* Contact with the eyes should be avoided during application.

# Price Relationships

## HOW TO USE THIS TABLE

WE HAVE INCLUDED this table to give you a sense of the relative costs of medications. Your actual price will vary considerably. Chapter 4 discusses the basis for the wide fluctuations in the costs you will encounter in your community.

For each medication we have included the approximate *wholesale* cost to the pharmacist of a *one day supply* of medicine. For topical or inhaled preparations we have included the *wholesale* cost of a customarily dispensed amount. Except where otherwise specified we have included the cost of a liquid preparation. For some preparations more than a dozen manufacturers supply the product; we have listed a middle price.

To estimate your cost you should multiply by the number of days' worth of medicine purchased and then calculate mark-up price in one of two ways commonly used: add $3.00 to the price, or divide the price by .6. For example, 10 days of medicine costing the pharmacist .36 a day will be .36 x 10 = $3.60. Adding $3.00 will make your cost $6.60; dividing by .6 would make your cost $6.00. Remember, these are only *rough* estimates of what you can expect to pay. Nevertheless, the prices we list are relative and you can certainly expect to pay more for a product that costs your pharmacist a dollar for a daily dose than one which costs two cents.

**Price Relationships**

| Usage Category | Medication (Generic Name) | Brand Names | Customary Amount Dispensed | Approximate Wholesale Cost (daily dose) |
|---|---|---|---|---|
| **Allergies** | Brompheniramine | Dimetane, Symptom 3 | | $ .12 |
| | Chlorpheniramine maleate | Chlor-Trimeton, Histaspan, Teldrin | | .08 |
| | Diphenhydramine | Benadryl, Benylin syrup | | .08 |
| | Tripelennamine | PBZ citrate, PBZ-SR, Pyribenzamine HCL | | .42 |
| | Tripolidine | Actidil | | .46 |
| **Asthma** | Albuterol | Ventolin, Proventil | | .38 |
| | Albuterol inhalant | | | 2.95 |
| | Beclomethosone inhalant | Vanceril Inhaler, Beclovent | | 6.32 |
| | Cromolyn | Intal | | .78 |
| | Metaproterenol | Alupent, Metaprel | | .21 |
| | Metaproterenol inhalant | | | 4.08 |
| | Prednisone | Deltasone, Meticorten, Orasone | | .18 |
| | Terbutaline sulfate | Brethine, Bricanyl | | .23 |
| | Theophylline | Tablets and capsules: Theophylline, Bronkodyl, Elixophyllin, Slo-Phyllin, Somophyllin-T, Theolair, Theophyl, Theophyl-chewable | | .16 |

| Category | Generic name | Brand names | Value |
|---|---|---|---|
| | | ORAL SOLUTIONS: BRONKODYL: ELIXICON, ELIXOPHYLLIN, SLO-PHYLLIN, SOMOPHYLLIN THEOLAIR, THEOPHYL, THEOCLEAR, THEOSPAN — TIMED RELEASE TABLETS OR CAPSULES: SLO-PHYLLIN GYROCAPS, ELIXOPHYLLIN-SR, THEOLAIR SR, THEOPHYL-SR, SUSTAIRE, THEODUR | .72 |
| BEHAVIORAL CONDITIONS | Chloral hydrate | NOCTEC | .03 |
| | Dextroamphetamine | DEXEDRINE | .14 |
| | Diazepam | VALIUM | .28 |
| | Imipramine | IMARATE, SK-PRAMINE, | .12 |
| | | TOFRANIL, TOFRANIL-PM | .04 |
| | Methylphenidate | RITALIN | .40 |
| | Pemoline | CYLERT | .14 |
| COLDS: COMBINATION DRUGS | | ACTIFED | .26 |
| | | DIMETAPP | .19 |
| | | NOVAHISTINE | .28 |
| | | TRIAMINIC | .36 |
| COLDS: DECONGESTANTS | Oxymetazoline | AFRIN, DURATRON, ST. JOSEPH DECONGESTANT FOR CHILDREN | .15 |
| | Phenylephrine | CORICIDIN, NEO-SYNEPHRINE, SUPER ANAHIST NASAL SPRAY | .12 |
| | Phenylpropanolmine (tablet) | PROPADRINE | .02 |

**PRICE RELATIONSHIPS (CONTINUED)**

| Usage Category | Medication (Generic Name) | Brand Names | Customary Amount Dispensed | Approximate Wholesale Cost (daily dose) |
|---|---|---|---|---|
| | Pseudoephedrine | NOVAFED, SUDAFED, AFRINOL-SYMTOM 2 | | .22 |
| | Xylometazoline | NEO-SYNEPHRINE II, OTRIVIN HYDROCHLORIDE, SINUTAB LONG LASTING 4-WAY LONG ACTING, DRISTAN LONG LASTING, SINE-OFF ONCE-A-DAY, SINEX LONG ACTING | | .15 |
| CONSTIPATION | Docusate | COLACE, SURFAK, KASOF, DIALOSE | | .32 |
| | Glycerine suppository | | | .65 |
| COUGH | Codeine (tablet) | | | .25 |
| | Dextromethorphan hydrobromide | | | .16 |
| DANDRUFF | Selenium sulfide | EXSEL, IOSEL 250, SELSUN, SELSUN BLUE | 4 ounces | 1.60 |
| | Zinc pyrithone | BRECK ONE SHAMPOO, DANEX SHAMPOO, HEAD AND SHOULDERS SHAMPOO, ZINCON SHAMPOO | 4 ounces | 1.26 |
| DIAPER RASH | A & D ointment | JOHNSON AND JOHNSON | 2 ounces | .70 |
| | Baby powder | BABY POWDER, BALMEX BABY POWDER, DIAPERENE BABY POWDER, FORMULA MAGIC LUBRICATING BODY TALC | 4 ounces | .73 |

| | | | Size | Price |
|---|---|---|---|---|
| **DIARRHEA** | *Cornstarch* | | 8 ounces | .40 |
| | *Desitin* | | 1.25 ounces | .90 |
| | *Zinc Oxide* | | 1 ounce | .60 |
| | *Diphenoxylate hydrochloride with atropine* | Colinil, Lomotil | 2 ounces | 3.83 |
| | *Kaolin/pectin* | | 8 ounces | 1.19 |
| | *Electrolyte and fluid replacements* | Lytren, Pedialyte | 32 ounces | 1.69 |
| **EAR** | *Acetic and ear solution* | Orlex Otic, VoSol Otic, Otic Domeboro Solution | 16 ounces | 3.35 |
| **EYE** | *Sulfacetamide* | Bleph-10, Cetamide, Sodium Sulamyd, Sulfacel-15, Vasosulf | | .17<br>.17 |
| **FEVER** | *Acetaminophen* | Liquiprin, Phenaphen, Tempra, Tylenol, Datril | | .11 |
| | *Aspirin* | Ascriptin, Bayer, Bufferin | | .08 |
| **FUNGAL INFECTIONS** | *Clotrimazole* | Lotrimin, Gyne-Lotrimin, Mycelex, Mycelex-G | ½ ounce | 4.50 |
| | *Griseofulvin (tablet)* | Fulvicin P/G, Fulvicin-V/F, Grifulvin V, Grisactin, Gris-PEG | | .48 |
| | *Haloprogin* | Halotex | 1 ounce | 12.45 |
| | *Miconazole* | MicaTin, Monistat-Derm (topical), Monistat 7 (intravaginal) | 15 grams | 2.41 |
| | *Nystatin* | Mycostatin, Nilstat, O-V Statin, Candex | 15 grams | 3.00 |
| | *Tolnaftate* | Aftate, Tinactin | 15 grams | 3.00 |

PRICE RELATIONSHIPS (CONTINUED)

| Usage Category | Medication (Generic Name) | Brand Names | Customary Amount Dispensed | Approximate Wholesale Cost (daily dose) |
|---|---|---|---|---|
| INFECTIONS (ANTIBIOTICS) | Amoxicillin | AMOXIL, POLYMOX, ROBAMOX, SUMOX, UTIMOX, WYMOX, TRYMOX | | .65 |
| | Ampicillin | AMERIL, AMPL-CO, D-AMP, DIVERCILLIN, PEN-A, PENBRITTEN, PENSYN, POLYCILLIN, PRINCIPEN, SARAMP, SK-AMPICILLIN, SUPEN, TOTACILLIN | | .42 |
| | Cefaclor | CECLOR | | 1.50 |
| | Cloxacillin | CLOXAPEN, TEGOPEN | | 1.12 |
| | Dicloxacillin | DYNAPEN, PATHOCIL, VERACILLIN, DYCILL | | .94 |
| | Eryhromycin | E-MYCIN, ILOTYCIN, ROBIMYCIN, RP-MYCIN, ILOSONE, E.E.S, PEDIAMYCIN, BRISTAMYCIN, ERYTHROCIN STEARATE, ERYPAR, ETHRIL, PFIZER-E, A/T/S, ERYDERM, STATICIN | | .60 |
| | Isoniazid | INH, NYDRAZID | | .03 |
| | Nitrofuratoin | CYANTIN, FURADANTIN, MACRODANTIN | | 1.01 |

| Generic | Brand names | Amount | Price |
| --- | --- | --- | --- |
| *Penicillin* | FALOPEN, G-RECILLIN, HYLENTA, KESSO-PEN, NOVOPEN-G, P-SO, PENLORAL, PENTIDS, PFIZERPEN, SK-PENICILLIN-G, SUGRACILLIN, BETAPEN-VK, COMPOCILLIN-VK, LEDERCILLIN VK, NADOPEN-V, PENAPAR VK, PVFK, REPEN VK, ROBICILLIN VK, SK-PENICILLIN VK, VITICILLIN VK, V-CILLIN K, VC-K, VEETIDS | | .25 |
| *Sulfisoxazole* | GANTRISIN, LIPO-GANTRISIN, SK-SOXAZOLE, J-SOL, ROSOXOL, SULFALAR | | .50 |
| *Tetracycline* | ACHROMYCIN, ACHROMYCIN V, BRISTACYCLINE, CENTENT, CYCLOPAR, TETRACHEL, T-250, FED-MYCIN, TETRACYCN, RETOT, ROBITET, ROY-CYCLINE, SK-TETRACYCLINE, SUMYCIN, TETREX | | |
| *Trimethoprim/ sulfamethoxazole* | BACTRIM, SEPTRA | | .14 |

**INFESTATIONS**

| Generic | Brand names | Amount | Price |
| --- | --- | --- | --- |
| *Crotamiton* | EURAX | 2 ounces | 2.88 |
| *Gamma benzene hexachloride (lindane)* | KWELL, GBH | 2 ounces | 2.20 |
| *Metronidazole* | FLAGYL | | 1.67 |
| *Pyrethins* | A-200 PYRINATE, BLUE RID, TRIPLE X, TISIT, TISIT | 2 ounces | 3.69 |

**INFLAMMATION**

*Steroids*
*Class I*

| Generic | Brand names | Amount | Price |
| --- | --- | --- | --- |
| *Halcinonide 0.1%* | HALOG | 15 grams | 3.55 |
| *Fluocinonide 0.05%* | LIDEX, TOPSYN | 15 grams | 3.84 |

**PRICE RELATIONSHIPS (CONTINUED)**

| Usage Category | Medication (Generic Name) | Brand Names | Customary Amount Dispensed | Approximate Wholesale Cost (daily dose) |
|---|---|---|---|---|
| | *Class II* | | | |
| | *Betamethasone valerate ointment/ lotion 0.1%* | VALISONE | 15 grams | 3.23 |
| | *Class III* | | | |
| | *Flucinolone acetonide ointment 0.025%* | SYNALAR | 15 grams | 3.66 |
| | *Triamcinalon acetonide ointment 0.1%* | ARISTOCORT, KENALOG | 15 grams | 2.95 |
| | *Fluranerenolide ointment* | CORDRAN | 15 grams | 2.95 |
| | *Class IV* | | | |
| | *Flucinolone acetonide cream 0.025%* | SYNALAR | 15 grams | 3.66 |
| | *Triamcinalone acetonide cream 0.1%* | KENALOG | 15 grams | 3.35 |
| | *Triamcinalone acetonide lotion 0.025%* | | 15 grams | 1.91 |
| | *Class V* | | | |
| | *Desonide cream 0.05%* | TRIDESILON | 1 ounce | .80 |
| | *Flumethasone pivalate cream 0.03%* | LOCORTEN | 15 grams | 2.72 |

| | | Quantity | Price |
|---|---|---|---|
| **Class VI** | | | |
| Hydrocortisone 1% | | 30 grams | .80 |
| **ITCHING** | | | |
| Aluminum acetate solution | BURROW'S SOLUTION, DOMEBORO, BLUBORO, ALUWETS | 16 ounces | 3.35 |
| Calamine lotion | | 16 ounces | 4.00 |
| Cyproheptadine | PERIACTIN | 16 ounces | .36 |
| Hydroxyzine | ATARAX, VISTARIL | | .91 |
| **PAIN** | | | |
| Acetaminophen | LIQUIPRIN, PHENAPHEN, TEMPRA, TYLENOL, DATRIL | | .11 |
| Aspirin (tablets) | ASCRIPTIN, BAYER, BUFFERIN | | .08 |
| Codeine | | | .25 |
| **SEIZURES** | | | |
| Ethosuximide | ZARONTIN | | .55 |
| Phenobarbital | ESKABARB, LUMINAL | | .07 |
| Phenytoin (tablet) | DILANTIN | | .07 |
| **SKIN: ACNE** | | | |
| Benzoyl peroxide | BENOXYL 5, 10, BENZAC 5, 10, 5 BENZAGEL, 10 BENZAGEL, DESQUAM-X 5, 10, LOROXSIDE, OXY 5, 10, PERSA-BEL, PERSADOX-HP, TOPEX, VANOXIDE, XERAC BP5, 10 | 1 ounce | 3.45 |
| Erythromycin-topical | A/T/S, ERYDERM, STATICIN | | |
| Sulfa/resorcinol | | 1 ounce | 3.00 |
| Tetracycline | ACHROMYCIN, ACHROMYCIN V, BRISTACYCLINE, CENTENT, CYCLOPAR, TETRACHEL, T-250, FED-MYCIN, G-MYCIN, MAYTREY, PALTET, PANMYCIN, TETRACYCN, RETOT, ROBITET, ROY-CYCLINE, SK-TETRACYCLINE, SYMYCIN, TETREX | | .14 |

PRICE RELATIONSHIPS (CONTINUED)

| Usage Category | Medication (Generic Name) | Brand Names | Customary Amount Dispensed | Approximate Wholesale Cost (daily dose) |
|---|---|---|---|---|
| | *Tetracycline-topical* | TOPICYCLINE | 1 ounce | 2.40 |
| | *Tretinoin* | RETIN-A | ½ ounce | 7.00 |
| SUNBURN | *PABA* | | 4 ounces | 4.00 |
| SWIMMERS' EAR | *Acetic acid solution* | ORLEX OTIC, VOSOL OTIC, OTIC DOMEBORO SOLUTION | 16 ounces | 3.35 |
| | *Acetic acid solution with hydrocortisone* | | 5 cc | 1.10 |
| VITAMIN A, C, D SUPPLEMENT | *Fer-in-sol iron* | FEOSOL, FER-IN-SOL, FERO-GRADUMET, MOL-IRON | 50 ml (drops) | 3.08 |
| | *Tri-vi-sol* | TRI-VI-SOL | 50 ml (drops) | 3.34 |
| VOMITING | *Prochlorperazine* | COMPAZINE | | |
| | *Emetrol* | | 10 ounces | .29 |
| | *Trimethobenzamide* | TIGAN | | 6.69 |
| | | | | .38 |
| WARTS | *Salicylic acid/ lactic acid mixture* | DUOFILM, SALACTIC FILM | 15 grams | 3.21 |
| WORMS | *Mebendazole* | VERMOX | | |
| | *Pyrantel pamoate* | ANTIMINTH | | .73 |
| | *Quinacrine* | ATABRINE | | .13 |

# Index